Nutrition and Addiction

a handbook

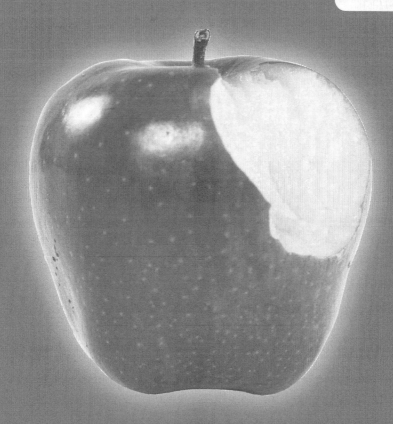

SUPPORTING RECOVERY FROM FOOD AND
SUBSTANCE MISUSE WITH NUTRITIONAL
AND LIFESTYLE INTERVENTIONS

Edited by Martina Watts

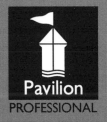

Pavilion
PROFESSIONAL

Nutrition and Addiction

A handbook

SUPPORTING RECOVERY FROM FOOD AND SUBSTANCE MISUSE WITH
NUTRITIONAL AND LIFESTYLE INTERVENTIONS

© Martina Watts (2011)

The authors have asserted their rights in accordance with the Copyright,
Designs and Patents Act (1988) to be identified as the authors of this work.

Published by:
Pavilion Publishing (Brighton) Ltd
Richmond House
Richmond Road
Brighton
BN2 3RL
Tel: 01273 623222
Fax: 01273 625526
Email: info@pavpub.com

Published 2011

*Pavilion Professional is an imprint of Pavilion Publishing, which aims to
address the issues important to higher level professionals and academics.*

A catalogue record for this book is available from the British Library.

ISBN: 978-1-908066-19-0

*Pavilion is the leading training and development provider and publisher in the
health, social care and allied fields, providing a range of innovative training
solutions underpinned by sound research and professional values. We aim to
put our customers first, through excellent customer service and value.*

Editor: Martina Watts
Production editor: Catherine Ansell-Jones, Pavilion
Cover design: Emma Garbutt, Pavilion
Page layout and typesetting: Tony Pitt, Pavilion
Printing: Charlesworth Press

Contents

Disclaimer

This handbook aims to provide general nutritional advice but is not intended to be a substitute for professional health advice. Always consult an appropriate health professional about any specific medical problems and keep them informed of any changes. Please note that sudden withdrawal from alcohol, opiates and tranquilisers may lead to serious (in the case of alcohol potentially fatal) withdrawal symptoms and requires close medical supervision.

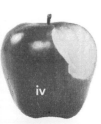

Nutrition and Addiction: A handbook © Pavilion Publishing (Brighton) Ltd 2011

Foreword

Joseph R Hibbeln, Captain in the United States Public Health Service

It is clear that, in one sense, we are all addicted to food. Without it we suffer a protracted period of withdrawal characterised by behavioural changes, craving for the substance, affective disturbances and ultimately, if the withdrawal is not treated, death. We anticipate the rewarding properties of food; we acquire it, ingest it and enjoy it, but crucially, unlike true addicts, we also inhibit this process wilfully or automatically so that at some point we stop eating, our appetites satiated.

One critical feature common to substance abuse and food addiction pathologies may be the failure of wilful or automatic control of these rewarding patterns of behaviour. How then does our nervous system integrate the complexities of the cultural meaning of food; the advertising and economics of food presentation; nutrient composition and amount; the immune, neuronal and neuroendocrine responses to food; the genetic diversity of response and the regulation of food behavioural patterns that are mediated by reward and disgust; all of which ultimately result in making choices about what foods to eat and when to stop eating them? We are clearly only beginning in our attempts to understand complex systems and how best to intervene. This book shares in the opening of this new field of research.

Critical questions emerge as to how the direct nutrient composition of these foods might affect the behavioural patterns of food anticipation and impulse regulation. For example, does sugar have direct feedback effects on the brain, acting as a neurotransmitter precursor, or are these feedbacks mediated by secondary homeostatic mechanisms such as insulin, leptin, adiponectin and ghrelin? Are some people so exquisitely sensitive to the rewarding properties in chocolate-containing foods that anticipatory behaviours in the seeking and acquisition of chocolate override all other social interactions? Do deficiencies in long chain omega-3 fatty acids

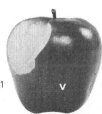

result in functional deficiencies in dopamine neural pathways underlying dopamine deficiency syndromes and result in endocannabinoid system hyperactivity, causing unregulated satiety?

The potential role of deficiencies in long chain omega-3 fatty acids, and excess consumption of omega-6 fatty acids has long interested me because these nutrients directly change the composition of the brain and result in a multitude of neurochemical, neurophysiological, behavioural and gene expression changes that are potentially concordant with the neural pathway changes that characterise addiction. Perhaps, most critically, the ingestion of addictive substances such as alcohol and tobacco can directly lower brain compositions of the long chain omega-3 fatty acid docosahexaenoic acid via peroxidation. How do these highly unsaturated fats get replaced in the brain? Among the most fundamental of issues is the fact that omega-6 fats from seed oils are cheap and abundant in the modern food supply whereas sources of docosahexaenoic acid, which is specifically required for optimal neural function, are less likely to be available to people with addictive behaviours.

As we choose to move forward in this field of scientific inquiry we must be reasonably confident to think that it will ultimately work to restore nutritional status and improve addictive behaviours. When I talk to addicts, they tell me about their personal experiences and the transformations achieved by more selectively choosing what foods they pull from trash cans and shelter offerings: '*Doc, I used to just eat anything, half a cheeseburger, whatever was calories. I was bad, sickly like. Now I only eat them veggies and stuff and I'm doing a lot better. Even got a job now*'.

An eloquent voice from the past is that of Macpherson Lawrie, a 20th century physician from the east end of London. In 1936, he wrote in *Nature Hits Back* that: '*In our whole endeavour to build up character and conduct, there is nothing more important than to appreciate the truth that physical nutrition is a psychological influence of the fundamental moment, an influence which, properly applied, not only prevents the appearance of much unpleasantness, contrariness and wrongfulness, but which directly and clearly liberates and fosters tolerance, agreeableness and kindness, friendliness and smiles.*'

Reference

Macpherson L (1936) *Nature Hits Back*. London: Methuen & Co.

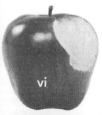

Contributors

Michael Ash BSc (Hons) DO, ND, F.DipION is an osteopath, naturopath and nutritional therapist. For over 25 years he worked in full-time practice, building one of the largest integrative health clinics in southwest England. After selling his clinic in 2006 and retiring from full-time practice in 2007, he has continued in his role as managing director of Nutri-Link Ltd, and as editor of www.nleducation.co.uk. He also writes and lectures and is developing novel therapeutic strategies for complex health problems through, where possible, the non-pharmacological manipulation of the mucosal immune system and its bacterial and other inhabitants. Michael was an early adopter of the principles and practices of functional medicine, directing his clinical practice to reflect these ideals from the early 1990s. His writing and developmental work embody these concepts.

Oscar Umahro Cadogan is a recognised authority on dietary and nutritional interventions for treating disease, natural sports nutrition, product quality and functional medicine laboratory testing in Denmark. He lectures extensively to practitioners and educational institutions and was a technical editor for the *International Textbook of Functional Medicine*, which is a comprehensive textbook on functional medicine. He works as a consultant in the health sector on research, legislation and the formulation of products and natural functional foods for the European and North American markets. He has published a range of healthy cookbooks, a book about natural treatments for serious gastrointestinal disease and is a regular contributor to both general media and professional publications in Scandinavia. He has seen thousands of patients one-to-one over the last decade and led multi-faceted health projects in some of Scandinavia's largest corporations.

Antony J Haynes BA (Hons) DipION BANT NTCC has been practising privately for over 19 years as one of the most experienced nutritional therapists in the UK, and is one of the first to implement the principles of functional medicine. He employs his clinical experience in managing the nutritional needs of his patients, which number in excess of 11,500, at his clinic in Harley Street, London. Antony is also head of technical services at

Nutri-Link, responsible for the technical and practitioner support team, as well as providing technical support directly to practitioners. For over 14 years he has been presenting clinically-focused workshops, lectures and seminars. He is also an award-winning author of two books on nutrition, *The Insulin Factor* and *The Food Intolerance Bible*, and has appeared on television and radio. In 2011, Antony was awarded the prestigious Complementary and Alternative Medicine award for Outstanding Practice for his many years of educating, inspiring and motivating practitioners and patients.

CAPT Joseph R Hibbeln MD is Acting Chief of Section of Nutritional Neurosciences, Laboratory of Membrane Biophysics and Biochemistry, National Institute on Alcohol Abuse and Alcoholism at the National Institutes of Health, Bethesda, Maryland. Joseph originated the field of omega-3 fatty acid deficiencies in affective disorders, contributing more than 80 peer-reviewed scientific papers. His research interests encompass severe pathological states, including suicide and psychosis, to normative personality in adulthood and early development. He believes that a substantial proportion of emotional distress in modern society might be reversed by adequate intakes of omega-3 fatty acids. His numerous honours include the TL Cleave Award from the McCarrison Society, London, United States Public Health Service (USPHS), Outstanding Service medal, three USPHS Crisis Response Awards, the Gerald Klerman award from the National Association for Research in Schizophrenia and Depression, Independent Investigator and Young Investigator awards from NARSAD and Eagle Scout, BSA. Dr Hibbeln received a BA with special honours from the University of Chicago in 1983 and an MD from the University of Illinois at Chicago in 1988. He is a board certified physician in psychiatry and serves as a Captain in the USPHS.

Yvonne Luna MA is a writer, performer and photographer who uses computer presentations to convey her experiences and views on social mores and mental health. Uncompromisingly honest, and often hilariously funny, Yvonne has been involved in award-nominated work, and has made presentations for conferences on the link between addiction, nutrition and mental health. She has been around the globe several times, though admittedly this was only because she couldn't find the entrance. She lives in Brighton, where she swims in the sea every day of the year, and catches her own mackerel by 'swishing' (swimming with a homemade bamboo swishing rod).

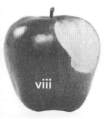

Jane Nodder MSc Nut Med BA(Hons) DipION NTCC is a practising nutritional therapist and senior lecturer and clinic supervisor for the BSc (Hons) in Complementary Medicine (nutritional therapy), in the School of Life Sciences at the University of Westminster, London. Her special interests include functional sports nutrition and nutritional approaches to weight management, eating disorders and endocrine modulation. Jane was a member of the National Institute for Clinical Excellence (NICE) Guideline Development Group for eating disorders from 2002–2004. She has recently completed an MSc in Nutritional Medicine at the University of Surrey, where her research study focused on dietary practices and nutritional knowledge in marathon runners. She has attended the Institute for Functional Medicine (IFM) intensive training programmes on 'Applying functional medicine in clinical practice' and 'Applying functional nutrition for chronic disease prevention and management' in the USA. Currently a member of the Council of the British Association for Applied Nutrition and Nutritional Therapy (BANT), Jane was previously chair of the BANT Professional Practice Committee. In 2010, she was awarded the Complementary and Alternative Medicine (CAM) award for Individual Excellence in Nutritional Knowledge.

Dr Alexandra J Richardson DPhil (Oxon) PGCE is a senior research fellow at the University of Oxford, a founder director of the UK charity Food and Behaviour (FAB) Research (www.fabresearch.org), and a leading expert on the role of omega-3 fatty acids in behaviour, learning and mood. She carried out the first controlled treatment trials of omega-3 for behaviour and learning in neurodevelopmental conditions such as ADHD, dyslexia and dyspraxia, played a key role in early research into omega-3 for adult psychiatric disorders, and currently has more than 90 research publications in peer-reviewed journals and academic books. Her ongoing research includes experimental studies and controlled nutritional treatment trials in both children and adults, and collaborations on several large scale multidisciplinary research programmes investigating the epidemiology of both neurodevelopmental and psychiatric disorders. She is also the author of *They Are What You Feed Them*, which provides practical dietary advice and an accessible summary of the scientific evidence that nutrition affects children's mental development and performance, with all author royalties dedicated to FAB.

Dr Marcus Roberts is director of policy and membership at DrugScope, the UK's leading independent centre of information and advice on drugs, and the national membership organisation for the drug field. From 2006 to April 2008, he was head of the policy and parliamentary unit at Mind, a charity that campaigns for better mental health. Marcus joined Mind in September 2006. Previously, he was head of policy at DrugScope and policy manager at Nacro, the crime reduction charity. He also worked at the Children's Legal Centre at the University of Essex. He was editor of the legal journal *ChildRight* from 1998 to 2000, and of *Safer Society*, the journal of crime reduction and community safety, from 2000 to 2002. He was Baring Foundation Fellow in philosophy and human rights at the University of Essex in 1994, and before joining the voluntary sector he spent time teaching philosophy and politics at the universities of Essex and Brighton, and as an associate lecturer of the Open University.

Helen Sandwell MSc Nut Med BSc (Hons) ANutr is an independent registered nutritionist. Since completing her master's degree in Nutritional Medicine in 2005, she has specialised in working with organisations dealing with drug and alcohol treatment, homelessness, offenders and people with mental health problems. In 2010, she completed a major project with the Prison Service, developing a nutrition module for people undergoing drug treatment in high security prisons in England. She has worked with Food Matters for several years developing the *Fab! Food and Wellbeing Programme*, a flexible programme of workshops, training and resources for delivery in a variety of community settings. Helen is a contributing writer to *Drink and Drugs News* magazine. Her website is www.goodfoodandhealth.co.uk

Martina Watts MSc Nut Med BA (Hons) DipION is a BANT and CNHC registered nutritional therapist with a special interest in digestive, behavioural and immune conditions. She is a member of the Professional Advisory Board at FAB Research and a committee member of the McCarrison Society for Nutrition and Health. She also works as an independent nutrition consultant at www.thehealthbank.com providing training sessions for the private and third sectors on improving personal and organisational resilience and performance with nutrition science, most recently for the award-winning Fareshare Community Food network. Martina has worked with Brighton and Hove Council to improve school meals, and with staff at a secure unit for young offenders in Greater Manchester to implement a cost-effective and successful healthy eating project. She is editor of *Nutrition and Mental Health: A handbook* also published by Pavilion.

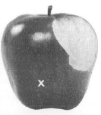

Nutrition and Addiction: A handbook © Pavilion Publishing (Brighton) Ltd 2011

Ann Woodriff Beirne has a BSc (Hons) in Food Science and an MSc in Applied Immunology. She worked for over 10 years in the NHS as a blood transfusion and haematology biomedical scientist before retraining as a complementary therapist. As well as having a busy practice in the UK, she worked as a lecturer in nutrition and immunology on the BSc (Hons) Nutritional Therapy degree course at the Centre for Nutritional Education and Lifestyle Management for seven years. She also worked as a sub-editor for the professional peer-reviewed journal, *The Nutrition Practitioner*, for three years before leaving to have a baby and emigrating to Australia. She is co-editor of the textbook *Biochemical Imbalances in Disease* and is currently working as a research supervisor for final year students' research projects at the Centre for Nutritional Education and Lifestyle Management.

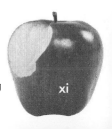

Introduction

Martina Watts

All addiction ends in pain

Addiction is a complex disease involving neurobiochemistry, drug chemistry and genetic, environmental and social factors. There are different levels of addiction, but the fundamental nature of it is the uncontrollable and compulsive craving, seeking and using of substances – even in the face of profoundly negative health and social consequences. This book examines the potential underlying nutritional and biochemical factors involved in addictive behaviour, and the importance of nutrition in the prevention and management of addiction. It also considers whether specific diet and eating patterns encourage addictive behaviour and consequent relapse rates, which remain alarmingly high. According to 2009/10 British Crime Survey data, in 50% of all violent incidents, victims believed the offender(s) to be under the influence of alcohol. In 20% of violent incidents, the victim believed the offender(s) to be under the influence of drugs. [1] Substance misuse in the workplace remains a significant cause of accidents, lowered productivity and absenteeism.[2]

Increasing evidence suggests that, alongside genetic, psychosocial and environmental factors, the chronic consumption of 'junk' food (in particular sugars and refined carbohydrates) is associated with food cravings and addictions. This behaviour may be a 'gateway' to other substances such as tobacco, alcohol and hard drugs. [3] The critical question to ask is whether our preference for such food is influenced by unconscious biochemical and addictive processes? In other words, does this 'choice' imply free will, or is it simply compulsive behaviour that we are hardly aware of?

1   Home Office Statistical Bulletin (2010) *Crime in England and Wales 2009/10.* London: Office for National Statistics.
2   Health and Safety Executive (2011) Drugs and alcohol at work [online]. Available at: http://www.hse.gov. uk/alcoholdrugs/index.htm (accessed 11 July 2011).
3   Avena NM, Rada P & Hoebel BG (2008) Evidence of sugar addiction: behavioural and neurochemical effects of intermittent, excessive sugar intake. *Neuroscience and Biobehavioural Review* **32** 20–39.

We have a genetic heritage that favours the craving of sugars which were historically rare and often difficult to access. Modern agriculture and manufacturing now permit the saturation of foods with sugars, yet we do not possess a mechanism that tells us when we have eaten too much of them. Our ancestral families lived for thousands of years in which excess was never experienced or anticipated, and we still carry their genetic legacy.

'Exporting' our dietary and lifestyle habits: a case of déjà vu?

I recall vividly the heat, sounds, smells and colours of a childhood in West Africa in the 1960s. My father, a civil water engineer, frequently took us on trips to source water supplies. I also remember that at each destination, no matter how poverty-stricken or remote, we would invariably find a cooler with soft drinks, supplied by multinational companies that had somehow managed to get there first. Finding chilled fizzy drinks in the poorest villages in the African bush seemed out of place and oddly inappropriate.

In developing countries, there has been a significant rise in the consumption of processed foods and soft drinks.[4,5,6,7] Excess sugar consumption has substantially changed the energy and structure of diets for many people.[8] Sugar has been replaced with artificial sweeteners in calorie-free diet drinks, yet artificial sweeteners are associated with weight gain, diabetes, taste distortion and an increased appetite for excessively sweet foods.[9,10,11] Calorie-dense meals containing refined carbohydrates,

4   Wasir JS & Misra A (2004) The metabolic syndrome in Asian Indians: the impact of nutritional and socio-economic transition in India. *Metabolic Syndrome and Related Disorders* **2** 14–23.

5   Hawkes C (2005) The role of foreign direct investment in the nutrition transition. *Public Health Nutrition* **8** 357–365.

6   Pingali P (2004) *Westernization of Asian Diets and the Transformation of Food Systems: Implications for research and policy. ESA working paper no. 04-17*. Rome: Food and Agriculture Organization of the United Nations.

7   Arroyo P, Loria A & Méndez O (2004) Changes in the household calorie supply during the 1994 economic crisis in Mexico and its implications on the obesity epidemic. *Nutrition Reviews* **62** 163–168.

8   Drewnowski A & Popkin BM (1997) The nutrition transition: new trends in the global diet. *Nutrition Reviews* **55** (2) 31–43.

9   Nettleton JA, Lutsey PL, Wang Y, Lima JA, Michos ED & Jacobs DR Jr (2009) Diet soda intake and risk of incident metabolic syndrome and type 2 diabetes in the multi-ethnic study of atherosclerosis (MESA). *Diabetes Care* **32** 688–694.

10   Fowler SP, Williams K, Resendez RG, Hunt KJ, Hazuda HP, Stern MP *et al* (2008) Fueling the obesity epidemic? Artificially sweetened beverage use and long-term weight gain. *Obesity* **16** 1894–1900.

11   Ludwig DS (2009) Artificially sweetened beverages. Cause for concern. *JAMA* **302** (22) 2477–2478.

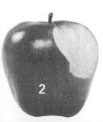

poor quality vegetable oils and low levels of fibre are increasingly preferred to traditional high fibre, low fat, low calorie diets.[12] At the same time, non-communicable diseases (including mental and neurological disorders) are becoming the dominant cause of ill health and are developing at faster rates now than they were in industrialised regions 50 years ago.[13,14]

By 2030 it is predicated that 298 million people in developing countries will have diabetes,[15] with complications from coronary artery and peripheral vascular disease, stroke, diabetic neuropathy, amputations, renal failure and blindness, reducing life expectancy and creating a substantial burden of health and other economic costs, which many countries cannot afford. The pace of social and technological change, and the rapid shift from pre-industrial, largely agriculture-based societies to modern urban industrial societies means that under- and over-nutrition may exist within the same household.[16]

Significant differences exist in the rates of obesity between rural and urbanised areas.[17] In rural areas, people are mostly lean and there is a lower prevalence of diabetes and heart disease. Those migrating to urban areas, however, are exposed to urbanised diets and lifestyles, and show greater rates of overweight and its associated risk factors.[18] Social and cultural influences are important factors, too, for in some countries large body size is associated with health and affluence.[19,20] So, another fundamental question to ask ourselves before inflicting modern convenience food and drink on our fellow man in Africa or Asia is: should we inform him that such products are potentially habit-forming, and that chronic consumption may lead to chronic health problems and, yes, a whole lot of pain?

12   Misra A, Singhal N & Khurana L (2010) Obesity, the metabolic syndrome, and type 2 diabetes in developing countries: role of dietary fats and oils. *Journal of the American College of Nutrition* **29** 3 (1) 289–301.

13   Popkin BM (2002) The shift in stages of the nutrition transition in the developing world differs from past experiences! *Public Health Nutrition* **5** (1) 205–214.

14   Watts M (Ed) (2008) *Nutrition and Mental Health: A handbook*. London: Pavilion Publishing.

15   Wild S, Roglic G, Green A, Sicree R & King H (2004) Global prevalence of diabetes: estimates for the year 2000 and projections for 2030. *Diabetes Care* **27** 1047–1053.

16   Popkin BM (2002) The shift in stages of the nutrition transition in the developing world differs from past experiences. *Public Health Nutrition* **5** (1) 205–214.

17   Popkin BM (2006) Global nutrition dynamics: the world is shifting rapidly toward a diet linked with non-communicable diseases. *American Journal of Clinical Nutrition* **84** 289–298.

18   Misra A, Sharma R, Pandey RM & Khanna N (2001) Adverse profile of dietary nutrients, anthropometry and lipids in urban slum dwellers of northern India. *European Journal of Clinical Nutrition* **5** (5) 727–734.

19   Brewis AA, McGarvey ST, Jones J & Swinburn BA (1998) Perceptions of body size in Pacific Islanders. *International Journal of Obesity* **22** 185–189.

20   Bhardwaj S, Misra A, Khurana L, Gulati S, Shah P & Vikram NK (2008) Childhood obesity in Asian Indians: a burgeoning cause of insulin resistance, diabetes and sub-clinical inflammation. *Asia Pacific Journal of Clinical Nutrition* **17** (1) 172–175.

The relationship between nutrition and addiction

This book focuses on nutritional approaches as fundamental therapeutic tools to complement traditional strategies for managing addiction. Leading researchers and nutrition practitioners explore the existing scientific evidence and newly emerging concepts alongside traditional strategies in the management of addiction. They also consider the role of stress, and the influence of genetic and environmental factors on our craving and reward systems, and discuss practical ideas for introducing safe, effective and evidence-informed nutritional programmes both in treatment centres and in the community.

Chapter 1 introduces drug policy within the UK, outlining the reasons why nutrition has so far not been part of drug and alcohol treatment, and why there is currently a better opportunity to incorporate fundamental nutritional principles than before. In Chapter 2, the biochemistry of the most relevant brain chemicals in addiction and dependency is explored, and diet and nutritional interventions proposed. The effects of nutritional deprivation on drug and alcohol users – and how they can be supported – is described in Chapter 3, with particular reference to the prison population.

Some people feel out of control around food and experience cycles of cravings and compulsive eating. Although the neurobiological evidence for food addiction is compelling, behavioural evidence is still lacking. Chapter 4 clarifies why there is still not quite enough evidence to classify food as an addictive substance. The historical, social and chemical factors behind chocolate – one of our tastebuds' most common objects of desire – are revealed in Chapter 5. As mentioned in the foreword, omega-3 fatty acids are critical for brain development and function. Chapter 6 expands on the role of dietary fats in addictive disorders and explains why our diet over the last 50–100 years is highly relevant in this context.

The science behind addiction is still in its infancy and novel (still controversial) connections are being proposed – some are discussed in this book. Chapter 7 hypothesises how food allergies may be involved in habitual, uncontrollable food cravings and how our food environment contributes. Chapter 8 considers the gut mucosal immune system as an increasingly important, yet often neglected area of mainstream healthcare,

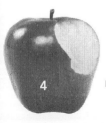

Nutrition and Addiction: A handbook © Pavilion Publishing (Brighton) Ltd 2011

and how our gut bacteria may be able to manipulate addictive tendencies and potentially help to resolve them.

The final chapter presents an engaging case history of how the choice of certain foods can affect mental health. Like most people, Yvonne was completely unaware that the treats she loved were capable of triggering an addictive process that profoundly affected her life. A dependence on any substance may become a vicious cycle as it biases our judgement (and potentially our biochemical pathways) towards maintaining the 'addiction', regardless of long-term consequences.

Unlike drugs, which are restricted and difficult to access, foods with 'abuse potential' are the most easy to access, the cheapest, least micronutrient dense and the most heavily advertised of products. Although scientists are still hotly debating whether or not being 'addicted' to food or drink resembles drug and alcohol addiction, we have to acknowledge that a significant number of people, when placed in specific environments, display behaviour that resembles addiction (such as bingeing, withdrawal and relapse). Furthermore, recent evidence from population-based and experimental animal studies suggests that pregnant women who eat high sugar/high fat diets are more likely to have children who are 'junk food junkies', with an increased risk of obesity and type 2 diabetes.[21,22]

For these reasons, protecting consumers with public health legislation does not seem excessive, such as regulating and taxing convenience foods and drinks high in sugar, fat and salt, and rigorously restricting the marketing of 'junk' food. In addition, and across all sectors in both developed and developing nations, nutrition and lifestyle education can help us further understand the relationship between what we consume and its effects on our health, and it can encourage us to change our behaviour. Starting is easy, but stopping is not.

---

21   Ong ZY & Muhlhausler BS (2011) Maternal 'junk-food' feeding of rat dams alters food choices and development of the mesolimbic reward pathway in the offspring. *FASEB Journal* **25** (7) 2167–2179.

22   Muhlhausler BS & Ong ZY (2011) The fetal origins of obesity: early origins of altered food intake. *Endocrine, Metabolic and Immune Disorders - Drug Targets* **11** (3) 189–197.

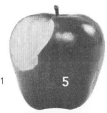

Chapter 1

Nutrition and drug treatment: an overview of drug policy

Marcus Roberts

Introduction

The principal focus of this chapter is the potential role of nutrition in the care and support of people who receive specialist treatment for drug misuse and alcohol dependency. It is argued that the issue of nutrition has been largely neglected in the development of drug and alcohol treatment, but that there are currently real opportunities to place it on the policy agenda.

Context and background

Neil McKeganey observed that 'the world of illegal drugs is a domain of truly staggering statistics' with the United Nations Office on Drugs and Crime estimating in 2007 that between 172 million and 250 million people had used illicit drugs worldwide in the last year.[1] For England and Wales, the best insight is provided in an annual report produced for the Home Office, *Drug Misuse Declared: Findings from the 2009–10 British Crime Survey*. It concluded that about three million adults in England and Wales used illicit drugs in 2009–2010, including about one million who had used Class A drugs. By far, the most widely used drug was cannabis, consumed by over two million respondents in the last year, followed by powdered cocaine, taken by about 800,000 people.[2]

---

1   McKeganey N (2011) *Controversies in Drugs Policy and Practice*. Basingstoke: Palgrave MacMillan.
2   Hoare J & Moon D (2010) *Drug Misuse Declared: Findings from the 2009–10 British Crime Survey*. London: Home Office.

It should be added that, according to the British Crime Survey, the level of illicit drug use in the last year was at its lowest level since recording began, mainly attributable to declining cannabis use since 2003–2004. It is also worth emphasising that the consumption of illicit drugs is much lower than the use of alcohol and tobacco. The Office for National Statistics reported in 2009 that around a fifth of adults in the UK were smokers.[3] In 2006, nearly three-quarters of men (71%) and over half of women (56%) had drunk alcohol at least once in the previous week.[4] The average consumption of alcohol in the UK had risen from five litres a year in the 1950s to 11 litres by 2007, with an estimated 10 million adults drinking in excess of the recommended limits.[5]

So when does drug use – legal or illegal – become a problem that nutrition might contribute to solving? First, it might be observed that, politically, substance misuse becomes a problem when it has an impact on the wider community – whether that is fears about the spread of HIV in the 1980s or concerns about drug and alcohol-related crime in the 1990s. Second, it is important to emphasise that most people who experiment with drugs do not use them in large quantities or over extended time periods, and after use, they move on with limited long-term impact on their health or well-being. Third, some drugs are more harmful than others, which is why drugs are classified as Class A, B or C under the Misuse of Drugs Act (1971) (with Class A drugs being the most harmful substances). A research study by Professor David Nutt and colleagues, published in *The Lancet* in November 2010, concluded that alcohol was the most harmful drug of all, followed by heroin and crack cocaine in second and third places.[6] These findings have sparked controversy, partly because the value of the whole scientific project of assessing the harmfulness of drugs in isolation and assembling them into league tables is open to challenge, not least given the increase in 'poly-drug use', typically involving the combination of alcohol and illegal drugs.[7]

3   Office for National Statistics (2009) Deaths related to drug poisoning in England and Wales. In: McKeganey N (2011) *Controversies in Drugs Policy and Practice*. Basingstoke: Palgrave MacMillan.

4   Smith L & Foxcroft D (2009) *Drinking in the UK: An exploration of trends*. York: Joseph Rowntree Foundation.

5   Institute of Alcohol Studies (2010) *IAS Factsheet: Alcohol consumption in the UK*. Cambridge: IAS. Cambridge and National Audit Office (2010) *Reducing Alcohol Harm: Health services in England for alcohol misuse*. London: The Stationery Office.

6   Nutt D, King L & Phillips L (2010) Drug harms in the UK: a multicriteria decision analysis. *The Lancet* **376** (9752).

7   A 2009 report from the European Monitoring Centre for Drugs and Drug Addiction (EMCDDA) concluded that '*in Europe today, poly-drug patterns are the norm, and the combined use of different substances is responsible for, or complicates, most of the problems we face*' (EMCDDA 2009, *Annual Report on the state of the drugs problem in Europe*). In September 2009, DrugLink, DrugScope's magazine, published its Annual Street Drug Trends survey, which concluded that '*younger, recreational users are now swapping or combining cocaine, ketamine, GHB, ecstasy, cannabis and alcohol as part of a night out*'.

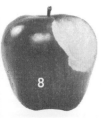

Another challenge is the constant emergence of new synthetic drugs, such as Spice and mephedrone (so-called 'legal highs'). Finally, a lot depends on patterns and forms of drug use – dependent drug and alcohol use is particularly harmful, so, for example, is injecting drug use.

A key point is that the most harmful patterns of drug and alcohol use are associated with other personal and social problems – people do not generally become dependent on heroin or crack cocaine without other problems, and drug and alcohol dependency will tend to have a devastating impact on their lives (and, of course, on families, partners and carers).[8] This does not necessarily preclude a neuro-scientific dimension. A recent research paper argued that *'addiction has a strong genetic component and both developmental stages (adolescents and young adults being at the highest risk for substance use dependency) and environmental factors (eg. exposure to stressful environments) play crucial roles in modulating the vulnerability for substance use dependency, in part through their influence on how the human brain works and responds, and adapts to various types of stimuli (including drugs).'*[9] But it has been the links between deprivation, social exclusion and drug dependency that have dominated recent research and policy, and rightly so.

As the first 10-year drug strategy, published by the Home Office in 1998, explained *'for older teenagers and people in their twenties, there are strong links between drug problems and unemployment, homelessness, prostitution and other features of social exclusion'.*[10] In 2006, the Advisory Council on the Misuse of Drugs (ACMD's) report *Pathways to Problems* concluded that *'from the late teens onwards, heavy smoking and problem drinking or drug use are strongly linked to socio-economic disadvantage,*

---

8   This does not mean that all the problems are concentrated in inner cities – former mining communities in rural areas were swept up in the heroin epidemics of the 1980s. Drugscope's magazine *DrugLink* recently reported on high levels of heroin use in the Shetland islands ('Heroin hinterland: The mysterious case of Shetland's young injectors', *DrugLink* **25** September/October 2010). There is some anecdotal evidence that 'legal highs' may have been more of a problem in remoter rural communities which lack established illegal drug markets. Poly-drug use is a phenomenon of the nighttime economy, which is socially mixed.

9   Volkow ND, Baler R & Goldstein R (2011) Addiction: pulling at the neural threads of social behaviours. *Neuron* **69**. This article continues: *'Scientific insights into drug-induced impairments of specific brain circuits are beginning to answer many of the questions that had baffled us for so long, such as (1) why drugs are so disruptive to social relationships, (2) why the social system users to deter behaviour (eg. the threats of incarceration or of loss of custody) does not work well in addicted subjects, (3) why social stressors (such as those that may be triggered by poverty) increase vulnerability to addictions… Ultimately, this leads to a cycle of drug abuse that is difficult to break free of, even when an addict may truly want to become drug free, resulting in the typical pattern of drug relapse so often seen in addicted individuals… Because the functions of these (brain) regions are also impaired in addicted individuals, this could explain an addict's inability to accurately steer their behaviours in appropriate directions despite having access to the required knowledge'.*

10   Home Office (1998) *Tackling Drugs to Build a Better Britain: The Government's 10-year strategy for tackling drug misuse.* London: The Stationery Office.

*often with disastrous results. Multiple drug use and drug injecting are
common in disadvantaged communities, in many of which problem drug
use has become an inescapable feature of life.'* [11] Indeed, the overwhelming
majority of the 25,000 under 18s in specialist treatment have problems
with alcohol and/or cannabis, and are not dependent drug users in the
adult sense. Their substance misuse problems are inextricably bound up
with other problems in their lives – whether that is exclusion from school,
involvement with the criminal justice system, mental health issues or
family breakdown.[12] In so far as improved nutrition may have a role in
addressing some of these issues (say performance at school or mental
well-being), it can contribute to prevention and early intervention.

The remainder of this article is primarily concerned with specialist
treatment for adults. For much of the last 10 years, drug policy and drug
treatment has been predominantly focused on the so-called 'problem drug
user' who is defined as someone dependent on heroin and/or crack cocaine,
but this has begun to change recently, with a significant rise in the number
of people presenting to drug services with other problems, particularly
involving powdered cocaine.

A dog that has not barked

The theme of nutrition has been marked mainly by its absence from the
development of drug policy and treatment in the last decade or so. Successive
drug strategies from New Labour in 1998 [13] (updated in 2002 [14]) and 2008
[15] and the coalition government in 2010 [16] have omitted any reference to it.
This is perhaps not so remarkable in strategic documents mapping out broad
policy objectives, but it is echoed in the clinical guidance that has shaped
frontline practice too. The 128 pages of *Drug Misuse and Dependence: UK
guidelines on clinical management* contain only three references to nutrition.
The most substantial observes that *'drug misusers may suffer from poor*

---

11   Advisory Council on the Misuse of Drugs (2006) *Pathways to Problems: Hazardous use of tobacco, alcohol and other drugs by young people in the UK and its implications for policy*. London: ACMD.

12   For further discussion, see Roberts M (2010) *Young People's Drug and Alcohol Treatment at the Crossroads: What it's for, where it's at and how to make it even better*. London: DrugScope.

13   Home Office (1998) *Tackling Drugs to Build a Better Britain: The government's ten year strategy for tackling drug misuse*. London: The Stationery Office.

14   Home Office (2002) *Updated Drug Strategy 2002*. London: Home Office.

15   Home Office (2008) *Drugs: Protecting families and communities* London: Home Office.

16   Home Office (2010) *Drug Strategy 2010: Reducing demand, restricting supply, building recovery: supporting people to live a drug free life.* London: Home Office.

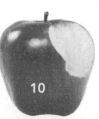

nutrition but should only receive oral nutrition support if there are clear medical reasons to do so. They should be given advice on diet and nutrition, especially if drinking heavily'. [17]

At the time of writing, the National Treatment Agency (NTA) was consulting on *Building Recovery in Communities* (BRIC), which will replace *Models of Care for Treatment of Adult Drug Misusers* (2002, updated in 2006) in attempting to set out a blueprint for treatment provision that reflects the best professional consensus and provides a good practice model for commissioners. [18] Nutrition does not get a mention in the BRIC consultation document.

A review of the literature produced by independent organisations in Britain tells a similar story. The author admits that DrugScope has had very little to say on nutrition and nor, to his knowledge, have the UK Drug Policy Commission or Alcohol Concern addressed this issue at any length. A recent report from the Royal Society of Arts, *Whole Person Recovery: A user centred approach to problem drug use* (2010), which ran to 140 pages, made no direct reference to nutrition as a theme, although it did note that 16% of service users identified help with day-to-day living, including food, as a key support issue. It did discuss the development of a peer-led drop-in café called The Hub in Bognor Regis, although it was mainly viewed as a support and networking initiative, with no direct reference to nutrition as such. [19]

As far as the author can see, it is a similar story when it comes to research literature. When one types 'nutrition' into the search engine of the respected *Drug and Alcohol Findings* website it turns up only nine articles, none of which are primarily concerned with nutrition. The two key guidance documents on drug misuse from the National Institute of Health and Clinical Excellence (on 'opioid detoxification' and 'psycho-social interventions' respectively, both published in July 2007) make no reference to nutrition. [20] The issue is, however, covered in recent NICE guidelines on alcohol. *Alcohol Use Disorders: Physical complications* (June 2010) makes clear that malnutrition is a condition associated with chronic alcohol

---

17   Department of Health, Scottish Government, Welsh Assembly Government and Northern Ireland Executive (2007) *Drug Misuse and Dependence: UK Guidelines on Clinical Management.* London: NTA. (There are only two other references to nutrition in this document, on pages 81 and 91).

18   National Treatment Agency (2011) *Building Recovery in Communities: A consultation for developing a recovery-orientated framework to replace models of care.* London: NTA.

19   Daddow R & Broome S (2010) *Whole Person Recovery: A user centred approach to problem drug use.* London: Royal Society of Arts.

20   NICE (2007) *Drug misuse: psycho-social interventions (NICE Clinical Guideline 51), Drug Misuse – Opioid Detoxification* (NICE Clinical Guideline 52).

misuse, and includes sections on *'nutritional support for alcohol-related hepatitis'* and *'nutritional support for alcohol-related pancreatitis'*. [21] NICE guidance on alcohol disorders does not, however, suggest that diet and nutrition could have any direct role in the treatment of dependency.

On reflection, the virtual silence on nutrition is surprising. No one who has spent any time in a drug or alcohol treatment service can be in any doubt that poor nutrition is a problem for many service users, many of who are visibly emaciated and malnourished. This is partly a consequence of the impact of drug or alcohol dependency on appetite and digestion. It also reflects poverty and deprivation, and the consumption choices that are made by people who have been spending a lot of their money on drink or drugs. Some may lack skills to shop for and cook nutritious food, and/or lack anywhere suitable to prepare and consume it. Some have other health problems that impact on nutritional needs and well-being.

The silence on nutrition is all the more striking when contrasted with the growing interest in nutritional issues in other areas of health and social care. In mental health, for example, there has been a lot of work on 'food and mood' (for example, food and mental health was the theme of a campaign launched by the Mental Health Foundation (MHF) in 2007, and both the MHF and Mind have produced information resources on food and mood). [22] The process of preparing and eating food (and growing it too) can be the heart and soul of voluntary and community sector projects in mental health (for example, in local Mind associations). The needs of people using drug and alcohol services are not dissimilar from many clients of mental health services.

Explaining the silence

So what might be the principal reasons for this silence on nutrition? First, it is arguable that drug policy to date has not been sufficiently engaged with the general health, well-being and quality of life of service users affected by and/or recovering from drug or alcohol problems. In the 1980s, the focus was on the development of harm reduction initiatives like needle exchanges, primarily in response to HIV/Aids. This was a public health

---

21 NICE (2010) *Alcohol Use Disorders: Physical complications* (Clinical Guidance 100) at pp. 131ff (hepatitis) and pp. 168ff (pancreatitis).

22 The MHF resource is available at http://www.mentalhealth.org.uk/help-information/mental-health-a-z/D/ diet/, and the Mind guide to *Food and Mood* is at http://www.mind.org.uk/foodandmood/food_and_mood-the_ mind_guide

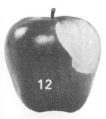

triumph, resulted in the lowest rate of HIV infection among injecting drug users in the world, and has saved countless lives, but it did not necessarily promote holistic engagement with the wider needs of service users. In the New Labour years, the investment of as much as £800 million annually in drug services dealing predominantly with 'problem drug users' (PDUs) with heroin and/or crack cocaine problems, was justified primarily by the crime reduction dividend. Research suggested that some PDUs committed a high volume of acquisitive crimes – such as shoplifting – to support their drug use. [23] Critics argue that the strong crime reduction focus of drug policy in this period resulted in too many service users being 'warehoused' on methadone, the opiate substitute, with too little additional support to move on and rebuild their lives. If drug treatment was narrowly focused in this way, there would be a tendency to neglect issues such as nutrition.

Second, the level of commitment to improving the overall health and well-being of any group of health or social service users (including their nutrition) will depend on the attitudes and perceptions of service providers, as well as the wider public, media and so on. Some mainstream health agencies, for example, may have different attitudes to people with drug and alcohol dependency problems to other patient groups, maybe because illicit drug use is illegal and both drug and alcohol dependency are widely viewed as 'self-inflicted'. At its crudest, some services may have a narrow focus on managing the 'addict', rather than picking up on and working to address other needs. Recently, there has been growing interest in the issue of 'stigma'. The UK Drug Policy Commission published a report called *Getting Serious about Stigma* in December 2010. While 59% of respondents to a public opinion survey saw drug dependence as an illness like any other long-term chronic health problem, 58% felt that *'one of the main causes of drug dependence is lack of self-discipline and will power'*. [24]

Third, there has been a marked pre-dominance of social modelling of the causes and contexts of drug and alcohol dependency in recent drug policy development. There is a strong evidence base for a relationship

---

23 Particularly influential was Christine Godfrey, Gail Eaton, Cynthia McDougall and Anthony Culyer (2002) *The Economic and Social Costs of Class A Drug Use in England and Wales 2000*. London: Home Office Research Study, which was more recently followed by Lorna Gordon, Louise Tinsley, Christine Godfrey and Steve Parrott (2006) *The Economic and Social Cost of Class A Drug Use in England and Wales 2003/04*. Home Office Online Report 16/06. This second study estimates the economic and social costs of Class A drug use to be around £15.4 billion in 2003/04, with drug-related crime costs accounting for 90% of costs associated with problematic drug use. A more recent, and detailed evaluation of the cost benefits of investment in the drug strategy can be found in National Audit Office (2010) *Tackling Problem Drug Use*. London: NAO.

24 UK Drug Policy Commission (2010) *Getting Serious About Stigma: The problem with stigmatising drug users*. London: UKDPC. See also Singleton N (2010) *Attitudes to Drug Dependence: Results from a survey of people in private households living in the UK*. London: UKDPC.

between drug problems and trauma and abuse, poverty and deprivation, homelessness, worklessness and so on, and there is a growing (and very welcome) emphasis on the importance of social (re)integration for recovery from substance misuse problems. It could plausibly be argued that a focus on social issues is less likely to encourage a close examination of the potential role of nutrition in the treatment of dependency itself than a more biological or neuro-scientific approach. Recent developments in the neuro-scientific research on drug use and dependency have been interesting, and may open up new opportunities for nutritionists to engage in clinical research and development. [25] Many of the problems associated with serious drug and alcohol problems – such as homelessness and poverty – will tend to compound problems with nutrition.

As a comparison, smoking cessation and tobacco-related harm is another health issue for drug and alcohol service users that has not been pro-actively addressed in many services. In a presentation to the National Drug Treatment Conference (2007), the smoking cessation expert Gay Sutherland claimed that *'most people in drug treatment smoke (between 70–90%) and are more nicotine dependent than the general population of smokers'*, with high rates of smoking among drug workers, too. Many drug services offer limited, if any, support for smoking cessation. In response to a 2008 consultation on the future of tobacco control, DrugScope commented that one possible reason for this limited involvement in smoking cessation was an under-development of health promotion. Drugscope commented that *'if health inequalities are to be narrowed then health promotion needs to be much more central to the work of frontline agencies working with the most socially excluded and marginalised. Drug treatment services could potentially learn from the sort of initiatives that have transformed mental health day service provision (for example, around healthy eating, exercise and interaction with the natural environment)'*. [26]

Breaking the silence

One of the triumphs of the past 10 years has been the adoption of an evidence-based approach to drug and alcohol treatment, with a growing recognition that people seeking help for drug and alcohol problems are

25 See World Health Organisation (2004) *Neuroscience of Psychoactive Substance Use and Dependence*. Geneva: WHO.

26 See DrugScope (2008) *Consultation on the Future of Tobacco Control: Response from DrugScope*. London: DrugScope.

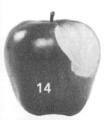

entitled to the same quality of care as all other patients receiving NHS funded health care provision. Those who believe that diet and nutrition can have a *clinical* role in the treatment of drug and alcohol problems will need to develop the evidence to support their claims. The relevant research is discussed by other contributors to this book and is not an area that the author is competent to comment on in any detail. The author would observe, however, that existing research on the role of nutrition in mental health or work with offenders (for example) will be relevant, given the substantial overlaps with substance misuse. For example, research has estimated that three-quarters of users of drug treatment services have a mental health problem, most commonly depression and/or anxiety (although 'more severe' problems like psychosis and personality disorder are not unusual). [27]

From a policy perspective, the next few years will see a truly radical transformation in the way drug and alcohol provision is planned, organised, commissioned and delivered. This will create a real opportunity to place nutrition firmly on the drug and alcohol policy agenda. Two developments are critical; first, the commitment to a 'recovery-orientated' approach to treatment and second, the transfer from April 2012 of around £1 billion of current drug and alcohol money to a new public health service.

Recovery

The emergence of recovery as an animating principle for drug policy in England might be traced back to the public debate that erupted in October 2007 in response to the publication of the National Treatment Agency's (NTA) annual report of that year. The numbers in drug treatment were continuing to rise, waiting times were falling and the majority of people who were starting treatment were staying engaged for the minimum 12-week period needed for it to have a positive impact – so far, so good. However, in a BBC interview the NTA's chief executive, Paul Hayes, was asked how many people were completing the treatment and coming out of it drug-free? According to the NTA's own figures, it was only around three per cent. On 31 October 2007, the *Daily Mail* complained about a '*£1.9 million bill to help just one drug addict kick the habit*' and *The Sun* declared that the '*NHS blows £130 million curing 70 junkies*'. David Davis, the then shadow home secretary, was prompted by the BBC coverage of the

---

27   See Weaver T, Madden P, Charles V, Stimson G & Renton A (2002) *Co-morbidity of Substance Misuse and Mental Illness Collaborative Study (COSMIC). Research summary.* London: NTA.

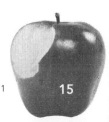

NTA figures to write to the chair of the House of Commons Public Accounts Committee asking for an investigation into drug treatment. '*This is an absolutely shocking revelation*', he declared, '*which speaks volumes about the government's competence and distorted priorities. It is yet more evidence why we should focus spending on getting addicts off drugs, and not just spend money managing their addictions*'. [28]

Unhelpfully, these responses viewed anything other than complete abstinence from drugs (including abstinence from – NICE recommended – substitute drugs like methadone) as treatment failure, and ignored the strides forward that had been made in improving the availability of drug treatment. However, as one commentator who was otherwise critical of what he dubbed '*The new abstentionism*' observed '*in some ways the BBC's intervention was a welcome return to forefronting what I'd guess most people think treatment should be about*', [29] a view of treatment that was being championed politically by the Conservative Party's Social Justice Policy Group. [30] When DrugScope launched a major consultation with its members and other key stakeholders in 2008, it found little support for a polarised debate that pitched 'abstinence' against 'harm reduction', as one contributor put it '*there is no "one size fits all" solution to the problems people who use drugs face*'. [31] The consensus was that we needed a balanced system – providing the right treatment, at the right time, in the right way. At the same time there was widespread concern that too many service users were being 'warehoused' on methadone, with too little expectation or aspiration for their recovery and re-integration.

Since 2007, a much richer understanding of what recovery does (and does not) mean has started to develop. In July 2008, the UK Drug Policy Commission published a report of the conclusions of its Recovery Consensus Group, which defined '*the process of recovery from problematic substance*

28   See Roberts M (2009) *Drug Treatment at the Crossroads: What it's for, where it's at and how to make it even better.* London: DrugScope.

29   Ashton M (2008) The new abstentionists. *DrugLink* Jan/Feb 2008. London: DrugScope.

30   Addiction Working Group (2006) *The State of the Nation Report: Addicted Britain.* London: Centre for Social Justice.

31   Roberts M (2009) *Drug Treatment at the Crossroads: What it's for, where it's at and how to make it even better.* London: DrugScope. See p26. It is worth quoting in full these comments from Sara McGrail, a freelance drug policy specialist: '*people experiencing drug treatment need the opportunity to choose the interventions that work best for them. This might change through someone's drug using career, with needle exchange, drop in, prescribing, inpatient and community detox and residential or community rehabilitation services coming into play at different points for different people. Sometimes, as we know, people will not move through these interventions in any convenient linear mappable way, but may well drift in and out of treatment over a protracted period of time. So is the aim abstinence? Yes. Is it maintenance? Yes. Is prevention important? Yes. There is no right or wrong answer and really there should be no debate about this. This is no "one size fits all" solution to the problems people who use drugs face*'.

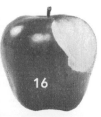

misuse' as *'characterised by voluntarily-sustained control over substance use which maximises health and well-being and participation in the rights, roles and responsibilities of society.'* The UKDPC explained that the requirement that recovery should *'maximise health and well-being'* encompassed *'both physical and mental good health as far as they may be attained for a person, as well as a satisfactory social environment'*. [32]

The definition of recovery that animated the 2010 Drug Strategy is informed by a similar vision. In the foreword to the strategy, the Home Secretary, Theresa May, declares that the solutions to drug and alcohol problems *'need to be holistic and centred around each individual, with the expectation that full recovery is possible and desirable'*. Recovery is identified with three overarching principles: *'well-being, citizenship and freedom from dependence'*. It is concluded that recovery is *'an individual, person-centred journey, as opposed to an end state, and one that will mean different things to different people. We must, therefore, put the individual at the heart of any recovery system and commission a range of services at the local level to provide tailored packages of care and support'*.

In November 2010 the Royal Society of Arts (RSA) published *Whole Person Recovery: A user-centred systems approach to problem drug use*, which discussed two RSA projects in West Sussex (Crawley and Bognor Regis), that aimed to place individual service users *'at the heart of any recovery system'*. The RSA described these projects as *'a catalyst for users themselves, and members of their communities, to foster recovery through their collective social effort and innovation'*. The report appealed to a *'theory of recovery capital'*, defined as the *'sum total of personal, social and community resources that someone can call on to aid their recovery'*, providing a *'more holistic model with which to spark and sustain recovery'*. [33] The RSA noted that this model of recovery communities accords with the current interest in localism and the vision of the Big Society.

This commitment to more recovery-orientated drug and alcohol treatment systems provides a clear opportunity to place nutrition on the drug policy agenda, both locally and nationally. If recovery is understood to require the maximisation of health and well-being, then the relevance of nutrition is unarguable, whatever its more direct role in treatment may or may not be.

---

32 It continued: *'The term "maximises" is used to reflect the need for high aspirations to ensure that users in treatment are enabled to move on and achieve lives that are as fulfilling as possible.'*
33 Daddow R & Broome S (2010) *Whole Person Recovery: A user-centred approach to problem drug use.* London: Royal Society of Arts.

Nutritionists must also make the case at local level for their role in recovery communities, including reaching out directly to service users. Locally, there will be a particularly strong case to be made for the potential for the cultivation, preparation and consumption of food as one of the core activities binding together recovery communities. Once nutrition has been placed on the recovery agenda in this way, it will create opportunities to examine whether it has a wider role in the treatment of drug and alcohol problems.

Public health

If the interest in recovery is an opportunity to raise the profile of nutrition within drug and alcohol policy, so too are the government's plans for the reform of the health service.

In April 2013, the National Treatment Agency will be abolished, with its key functions absorbed into a new public health service, Public Health England, which will control around £1 billion of current drug and alcohol service expenditure (around a quarter of the total public health budget). At local level, the commissioning of drug and alcohol treatment will be the responsibility of directors of public health. The directors of public health will sit on local statutory health and well-being boards, which will bring together the main public health, NHS and social care leaders to work together. The boards will have a responsibility for assessing and meeting the needs of the whole local population. At the time of writing, the proposed minimum membership of health and well-being boards will comprise elected representatives, GP consortia, directors of public health, directors of adult social services, directors of children's services, local health watch (which provides representation for patients) and, where appropriate, the new National Health Service Commissioning Board. There will be flexibility locally to expand the membership of these boards (for example, to include local voluntary groups). [34]

As a result of these reforms, drug and alcohol services will no longer be the responsibility of an NHS special health authority – ie. the National Treatment Agency – but will be integrated into the wider public health remit. It is currently proposed that Public Health England will also be responsible for the provision of services including health protection,

---

34   At the time of writing, the Government is consulting on these reforms through the Department of Health (2011) *Healthy Lives, Healthy People: Our strategy for public health in England* (white paper).

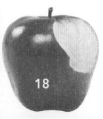

emergency preparedness, sexual health, immunisation programmes, obesity, smoking cessation, health checks, screening and child health promotion. Critically, Public Health England will have the lead responsibility for nutrition within government. This means that the new public health service will bring together responsibility for drug and alcohol treatment and nutrition within the scope of a single agency, and under the umbrella of the director of public health at the local authority level.

Conclusion

There has perhaps never been a more auspicious time to press the arguments for the potential role of nutrition in drug and alcohol treatment, as part of a more holistic and recovery-orientated response to the needs of people who develop serious substance misuse problems.

And there is a wider argument here too – about the impact of inequality on access to healthy food. People with drug and alcohol problems typically experience social exclusion and marginalisation – for example, poverty, worklessness and homelessness. (Their well-being is often also dependent on the nutritional provision that is available in institutional settings, including prisons and hostels). In the foreword to the public health white paper, *Healthy Lives, Healthy People*, the Secretary of State for Health, Andrew Lansley, identifies the desire to address health inequalities as one of the main drivers behind the public health reforms, acknowledging that *'health inequalities between rich and poor have been getting progressively worse'*, and declaring *'we cannot sit back while … so many people are suffering such severe lifestyle-driven ill health and such acute health inequalities'*. [35] Improving the nutrition of the most marginalised people in society, including people with drug and alcohol problems (and their families), has an important contribution to make to addressing these wider health inequalities. Where local directors of public health make progress in reducing health inequalities, they can benefit their areas financially through the proposed new health premium.

Marcus is director of policy and membership at Drugscope.

---

35 Department of Health (2011) *Healthy Lives, Healthy People: Our strategy for public health in England.* London: DH.

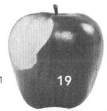

Chapter 2

Perspectives on the neurobiochemistry of addiction and implications for nutritional management

Oscar Umahro Cadogan

Introduction

Nutrition and nutritional therapy should be included in the mainstream management and treatment of addiction, not as the sole tool – or at the expense of interventions with a longer tradition, greater acceptance and a larger research base – but alongside standard interventions.

Drug addiction causes extensive changes in neurobiochemistry, cerebral blood flow, cerebral energy utilisation, neuronal signaling, neurophysiology and neuroplasticity. While a drug is active these changes are short-term but when a drug is used over a long period they can become permanent. This is the reason why drug addiction can be so difficult to break.

Nutrition can have an impact on neurobiochemistry, neuroplasticity, neuronal signaling and neurophysiology and these can be altered, improved or normalised with the help of nutritional interventions and nutritional therapy. As a result, there is a need for a more comprehensive use of nutritional therapy in the management and treatment of addiction.

Note: The terms 'addict', 'drug addiction' and 'drug abuse' are used in this chapter and other chapters. Some working in the field may prefer the term 'dependent substance user'. For further clarification on drug terminology, please refer to the **Drug terms** on page 186.

Mental illness and addiction

Mental illness is often, but not always, a major risk factor for becoming an addict – and drug addiction, in turn, can cause mental illness. There is increasing recognition that nutritional therapy can make a difference in the management of mental illness. Therefore, if for no other reason, nutritional therapy should be used in all cases with a dual diagnosis of mental illness and addiction.

Our knowledge of the impact of nutrition on neurobiochemistry from orthomolecular psychiatry also sheds light on various neuronal pathways and the synthesis of numerous neurotransmitters, which can be utilised in a more direct manner in the management of addiction.

The neurotransmitters dopamine, serotonin, noradrenalin, gamma-aminobutyric acid (GABA) and glutamate all play an important role in mental illness and addiction, as does neuroplasticity (explained in detail later in the chapter). Where nutritional therapy can be used to impact upon the alterations in the production, release, transport and re-uptake of these neurotransmitters, as well as neuroplasticity in mental disease, it may also be used to impact upon the same issues in addiction.

Addiction often leads to poor nutritional status and poor nutritional status affects mood and mental functioning. This is yet another reason to make nutritional intervention and therapy part of the management and treatment of addiction.

Neurotransmitters and neural pathways in addiction

To fully appreciate how nutrition can be used in the recovery from drug addiction and how it can help to prevent relapse, it is essential to know the workings of the key neurotransmitters and neural pathways and networks that are affected by drugs in the short and long-term.

Dopamine

Dopamine is one of the primary neurotransmitters in the structures, networks and pathways of the brain associated with reward, pleasure and well-being. Dopamine release plays a central role in the experience of pleasure and primes us to repeat a behaviour to acquire the reward in the future. It also helps us to focus and execute tasks because it is a dominant neurotransmitter in the neural networks and brain centres that play central roles in decision-making, inhibition, learning, balancing long-term goals with short-term gratification, and social conduct.

The roles of dopamine:

- learning
- reward
- focus
- executing tasks
- well-being
- pleasure
- behaviour
- cognition
- punishment
- attention
- mood
- sleep
- working memory
- movement.

Dopamine synthesis

Dopamine is synthesized from the amino acid L-tyrosine, which in turn can be synthesized from the amino acid L-phenylalanine. Dietary composition can affect dopamine production. By increasing the intake of protein and lowering the amount of carbohydrates consumed, the production of dopamine can be enhanced as more L-tyrosine will be transported across the blood–brain barrier when blood sugar and insulin levels are lower.

The velvet bean (Mucuna pruriens) contains significant levels of L-dopa, which is the immediate precursor to dopamine. Dietary supplements made with velvet bean extracts or concentrates might help stimulate dopamine synthesis by providing the immediate precursor.

Nutrients that are important in the production and metabolism of dopamine are:

- folate (vitamin B9)
- pyridoxine (vitamin B6)
- magnesium
- vitamin C
- copper
- iron
- zinc
- vitamin B12.

The dopamine transporter (DAT)

The dopamine transporter pumps dopamine out of the synapse and back into neurons. Following the use of cocaine, methamphetamine and certain other drugs that work in part by either blocking the dopamine transporter or making it function in reverse so that it empties neuronal stores of dopamine into synapses and causes excessive dopaminergic stimulation. Subsequent to the use of cocaine, methamphetamine and other drugs that interfere with normal dopamine transport, the depletion of neuronal stores of dopamine is likely, leading to decreased functioning in all neural networks where dopamine is an important neurotransmitter. Using nutritional support to increase dopamine production might help ameliorate some symptoms that are at least partially caused by a dopamine deficit after drug use, such as mood swings, impaired learning and impaired concentration.

Dopamine receptors

There are two major groups of dopamine receptors:

1. D1-like receptors
2. D2-like receptors.

Lower levels of D2-like receptors have been associated with an increased risk of drug use and of becoming addicted once using drugs and other stimulants. Furthermore, lower levels of D2-like receptors have also been associated with an increased risk of gambling addiction and other uncontrolled compulsive behaviours. Supporting dopamine synthesis and function with dietary changes in the ratio of protein to carbohydrates, supplementation with L-tyrosine and the co-factors important in the synthesis and metabolism of dopamine might help ameliorate some of the consequences of lower levels of D2-like receptors.

Noradrenaline

Noradrenaline is the primary neurotransmitter in the part of the brain called the nucleus coeruleus. The nucleus coeruleus plays an important role in alertness, the stress response and arousal. Arousal is defined as the state of being awake or reactive to stimuli. It is a condition of sensory alertness, mobility and readiness to respond. Arousal is important in regulating consciousness, attention, and information processing. It is crucial for motivation to act and for certain behaviours such as mobility, the pursuit of nutrition, the 'flight or fight' response and giving attention to a task. Thus when noradrenaline is released, the initial response is the ability to act, react and focus, but if the production is excessive, the response is stress.

The roles of noradrenaline:

- stress hormone
- attention and arousal (at lower levels)
- fight or flight response.

Noradrenaline is produced from dopamine. Consequently, all the nutrients and changes in diet that support dopamine production can also support noradrenaline production. Supporting the synthesis of noradrenaline might be helpful as a deficit of noradrenaline after the effect of a drug wears off is likely to be part of the reason for apathy, problems with concentrating, a lack of motivation and other symptoms.

Glutamate

Glutamate is one of the most abundant neurotransmitters in the brain. It is also one of the most tightly controlled neurotransmitters as an excess of glutamate causes rapid neuronal death. Glutamate is a neurotransmitter of key importance in addiction, both in relation to becoming addicted and in relation to interventions of benefit in managing addiction.

The roles of glutamate

Glutamate has several important functions in the central nervous system (CNS):

- it facilitates learning and memory

- it increases neuronal activity levels and sensitivity to all other inputs, signals, messenger molecules and stimuli

- it facilitates neuroplasticity and neuronal remodeling (essentially changing the connections between neurons and different parts of the brain)

- it causes neuronal apoptosis (programmed cell death) when secreted in excess, as excess glutamate stimulates the neuronal intake of calcium ions; once the concentration of calcium ions in a neuron reaches a certain level, the neuron undergoes apoptosis.

Glutamate and addiction

Glutamate is an important neurotransmitter in the nucleus accumbens – a brain region that plays a key role in addiction. Many substances of abuse will increase glutamate levels during the 'high', but subsequently there will be a glutamate deficit. The changes from excess to deficit impact the nucleus accumbens and may promote drug-seeking behaviour and relapse. Long-term, glutamate levels are decreased. Normalising glutamate levels decreases cravings and might help 'unlearn' drug-seeking behaviour. Blocking glutamate receptors prevents animals from becoming addicted to substances of abuse.

Glutamate synthesis and metabolism

Glutamate production is related to protein intake. Higher protein intake will normally result in higher levels of glutamate being available. Glutamate can be converted into the neurotransmitter gamma-aminobutyric acid (GABA), which has the exact opposite effect of glutamate. Rather than being an excitatory and stimulatory neurotransmitter, GABA is an inhibitory neurotransmitter. The conversion of glutamate into GABA requires the co-factors pyridoxine (vitamin B6) and magnesium. L-theanine, a component of green tea, also appears to enhance the conversion of glutamate to GABA. Under normal conditions, the ratio of glutamate to GABA is constantly regulated to achieve a perfect balance between alertness and activity (via glutamate) and neuronal inhibition to prevent hypersensitivity. If this delicate balance is upset, problems with hypersensitivity and neuronal death may occur.

Glutamate transport

Since glutamate has such a potent effect on neurons and neuronal functioning, the release and transport of glutamate is tightly controlled. Astrocytes (a type of cell in the central nervous system, distinct from neurons, whose role it is to help maintain the delicate biochemical environment in the brain) quickly release and remove glutamate to either stimulate or inhibit neuronal activity and neuroplasticity. Astrocyte functioning is therefore of major importance in regulating cerebral levels of free and active glutamate.

The glutamate cystine transporter

The glutamate cystine transporter works by pumping cysteine or cystine (both are sulphur-containing amino acids) into astrocytes, which then release glutamate at the same time. Sufficient levels of cysteine and cystine in the brain are important for adequate levels of glutamate to be released.

Cysteine is also necessary for the production of the molecule glutathione. Glutathione is an antioxidant produced by the body that helps protect against the damaging effects of excess glutamate, if release is not controlled properly. In short, cysteine is important when there is too little or too much glutamate.

Following drug use, glutamate release is usually insufficient, leading to decreased cerebral activity and decreased neuroplasticity. Since GABA is produced from glutamate, low or insufficient GABA might also be a problem once the effect of a drug wears off. These problems might be ameliorated by:

- providing the amino acid N-acetyl-cysteine (NAC) to increase the release of glutamate

- providing pyridoxine (vitamin B6) and magnesium to support the synthesis of GABA.

Serotonin

Serotonin is a dominant neurotransmitter in neural networks, centres and functions associated with the regulation of sleep and mood. Abnormal levels of serotonin and altered serotonin transport and signaling have been associated with mood disorders such as depression, obsessive compulsive disorder and more recently with addictive behaviours. Steps to normalise serotonin levels will sometimes, but not always, provide some benefit.

The roles of serotonin:

- circadian rhythm

- mood

- stress levels

- satiety

- hunger

- muscle contractions

- core temperature

- aggression

- sociability

- paranoia.

Serotonin (5-hydroxytryptamine or 5-HT) is synthesized from the amino acid tryptophan. Providing sufficient levels of the following nutrients important for serotonin synthesis and metabolism:

- folate (vitamin B9)

- pyridoxine (vitamin B6)

- magnesium

- vitamin C

- vitamin B12.

The immediate precursor to serotonin is 5-hydroxytryptophan (5-HTP). 5-HTP is produced from tryptophan but can also be supplemented pre-formed as an extract or concentrate of the seeds from Griffonia simplicifolia – a West African medicinal plant.

Endorphins

Endorphins are endogenous opioid peptides that function as neurotransmitters and resemble opiates in their ability to produce analgesia and feelings of well-being. Endorphins play a key role in the effects of drugs and in both creating a state of addiction and maintaining it.

The roles of endorphins:

- stimulate a sense of satiety

- decrease emotional and physical sensitivity to pain and discomfort

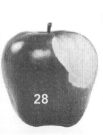

- decrease the mediation of pain signals

- elevate mood

- cause nausea in excess

- inhibit smooth muscle activity

- trigger the release of dopamine in neural networks and areas of the brain that play a key role in both reward and addiction.

Endorphin production can be affected by diet. Phenylethylamine found in cocoa can stimulate the release of endorphins, as can very rich and savoury foods and ingredients such as sugar, butter, cream, cakes, ice cream, sugary drinks and rich sauces. Most of these cannot be recommended to increase endorphin production as they are 'unhealthy' in excess and may destabilise neurobiochemistry. However, eating dark chocolate and cocoa, obtaining sweetness through fruits and increasing the intake of beneficial fats from fatty fish, nuts, seeds and cold-pressed unrefined vegetable oils are all viable options.

Drugs and neurotransmitters	
Cannabis	Contains tetrahydrocannabinol (THC) which targets cannabinoid 1 (CB1) receptors and glycine receptors
	CB1 receptor activation lowers the release of other neurotransmitters and decreases neuronal sensitivity
Cocaine	Blocks the dopamine transporter (DAT) leading to greatly increased levels of dopamine in various parts of the brain
	Blocks the uptake of dopamine, serotonin and noradrenaline via monoamine transporters
	Alters glutamate release in several brain centres
	Lowers glutamate in the nucleus accumbens
Ecstasy (MDMA)	Blocks the re-uptake of dopamine, serotonin and noradrenaline
	'Reverses' the transport of dopamine, serotonin and noradrenaline from removal to release, causing a decrease in sensitivity to the neurotransmitters due to overstimulation
	Stimulates serotonin receptors directly

continued over

Drugs and neurotransmitters (continued)	
Ethanol	Decreases glutamate release and functioning
	Stimulates GABA-A receptors
	Interferes with general neuronal functioning
Mephedrone	Promotes the release of dopamine, serotonin and noradrenaline and subsequently blocks their re-uptake
Methamphetamine	Increases levels of dopamine, noradrenaline and serotonin
	Activates reward circuitry
Opioids	Work by stimulating opioid receptors, leading to decreases in GABA and disinhibition of dopamine production, release and signaling

What do we know about the neurobiochemistry of addiction?

Reward circuitry

The brain's reward circuitry consists of neural networks and structures that:

■ 'reward' certain behaviour

■ control cravings

■ are involved in the sensation of pleasure

■ help promote/reinforce behaviours that trigger those networks.

Under normal circumstances, the reward circuitry is activated as a response to activities and events which are both pleasurable and beneficial, thus promoting and reinforcing behaviour of benefit to the person. Dopamine is recognised as a key neurotransmitter in these brain structures and neural networks. As a result, much of the neurobiochemical research on drug addiction (and addiction in general) has focused on dopamine.

Hereditary variations in the production of dopamine and the amounts and types of dopamine receptors can either increase or decrease the risk of becoming an addict. The variations leading to a lower dopamine production or decreased dopamine sensitivity increase the risk of addiction; the ones that lead to increased dopamine synthesis or increased dopamine sensitivity decrease the risk of addiction.

Supporting dopamine production, synthesis and sensitivity is therefore of major importance in the management of addiction and the prevention of relapse. There are several known dietary, nutritional and lifestyle interventions that can support the synthesis and transport of dopamine as well as help maintain dopamine sensitivity:

- omega-3 fatty acids
- supplementation with folate (vitamin B9) and vitamin B12
- supplementation with vitamin B6 and magnesium
- exercise
- supplementation with the amino acid N-acetyl-cysteine (NAC)
- supplementation with vitamin C and the trace mineral copper
- supplementation with the amino acids L-phenylalanine or L-tyrosine.

Rewiring of reward circuitry

When drugs are abused, reward circuitry is not only activated strongly and briefly while the drug is active, it is also changed and primed to make the addict seek out the drug repeatedly, even to their detriment. Other activities and triggers that would normally activate this circuitry are no longer able to do so, following the neurobiochemical and neurophysiological changes that have occurred in the brain as a result of drug abuse. As a result, abusing drugs becomes the addict's only or primary method of stimulating the brain centres involved in well-being, motivation and reward. This process is a vicious cycle.

Neuroplasticity

The human brain is quite capable of change and re-organisation. The neurobiochemical term for this is 'neuroplasticity'. Neuroplasticity is of major importance in the development of addiction and also in its treatment. In order to create new neural connections and break old ones, the neurotransmitter glutamate must be released, which facilitates neuronal reorganisation and increases neuronal activity. In short, glutamate helps to facilitate the 'rewiring' of the brain.

Most drugs will force a massive release of glutamate in various brain structures and neuronal networks while active, thus helping to 'rewire' the brain for addiction. After the effect of the drug wears off, glutamate production is often impaired; and once the brain is 'wired' to (re)seek the drug/substance of choice, those changes become extremely hard to break – even with the help of extensive psychosocial interventions. This occurs because of the changes at neurophysiological and neurobiochemical levels caused by the alterations in neuroplasticity.

For this reason, focusing on optimising and normalising glutamate production is of major importance in the management of addiction, to help promote more favourable neuroplastic changes. Increasing glutamate production at the appropriate time may make it easier to break the vicious cycle of addiction by enabling the reorganisation of neural networks that have been 'rewired' for addiction.

Breaking the cycle of addiction

If neuroplasticity can be enhanced as part of a treatment programme, then it may be more straightforward to break the cycle of addiction as it will be easier to form new neural pathways and disrupt previously created ones. In short, increasing neuroplasticity may facilitate the physical changes in the brain necessary for a long lasting change in behaviour (abstinence), which is the aim of most treatments for drug abuse.

As described in this chapter, neuroplasticity can be enhanced by changes in diet, lifestyle and nutritional interventions. Conversely, an unhealthy lifestyle and diet and substances of abuse reduce neuroplasticity.

Stress leads to use or relapse

Once addicted, stress can cause drug-seeking behaviour or relapse during abstinence. Stressful situations and pressure can also lead to the initiation of drug use and subsequent addiction. Avoiding stress is obviously of importance but as diet and lifestyle have a major impact on the activation of stress circuitry in the brain and the activation of the systemic stress response – and as stress sensitivity can be altered by lifestyle interventions – diet and nutritional therapy are useful tools for dealing with this aspect of relapse.

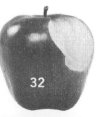

Adrenocorticotropin hormone and stress

The adrenocorticotropin hormone (ACTH) is released in the brain during stressful states and helps trigger the physiological stress response. The precursor to ACTH is proopiomelanocortin (POMC), a polypeptide. When ACTH is cleaved from POMC, some of the other fragments released are converted into endogenous opioids.

Is the link between stress and drug-seeking behaviour and/or relapse related to opioid signalling via POMC?

Previous addicts who start taking opioids such as morphine and heroin often relapse to full-scale addiction, even if they were originally addicted to another drug such as cocaine or cannabis. Stress also causes relapse. The link may be that during stress not only stress hormones are released, but also opioids. Could these 're-trigger' addiction?

Furthermore, the emotional responses to stress also lead to an increased urge to (re)use drugs as the drugs will help to decrease some of the uncomfortable emotional responses.

Nutrition affects the stress response

As nutrition affects the stress response, this is another reason for utilising nutrition in the management of addiction. Many aspects of typical modern foods serve to increase the stress response and the sensitivity to stress hormones. These include:

- high glycaemic loads, resulting in unstable blood sugar levels

- pro-inflammatory foods and food components may also trigger the stress response at the neurological level (eg. sugars, refined carbohydrates, heated vegetable oils with a high omega-6 to omega-3 ratio, trans fats, commercially produced meat high in omega-6, allergens that provoke inflammatory responses in individuals)

- alterations in gut flora as a result of insufficient fibre and phytochemicals and excess refined sugar, unhealthy fats, food additives and low-quality protein; changes in gut flora may affect serotonin production and initiate the stress response.

Fortunately, dietary changes and specific nutrients can help decrease the stress response and lower sensitivity to stress hormones. These include:

- omega-3 fatty acids from fish, flaxseed, flaxseed oil, walnuts, walnut oil, canola oil, game and organic animal products

- magnesium and potassium from green vegetables, nuts, seeds and wholegrains

- fibre and fibre-rich foods stabilise blood sugar levels, providing a feeling of satiety, and increase the production of cholecystokinin (a key digestive hormone)

- high quality protein stabilises blood sugar and provides an increased feeling of satiety.

Aspects of obsessive compulsive disorder?

Drug addiction and obsessive compulsive disorder (OCD) share several characteristics:

- people are compelled to act in specific ways that have no benefit or might even be detrimental

- they (almost) cannot resist the urge to engage in particular behaviours

- specific cues, memories, events and social situations can trigger compulsive behavior.

At times people may be aware of the issue but still unable to avoid the compulsive behaviour. At other times the behaviour will not be consciously noted as being a problem. Since there are similarities in the behaviour and characteristics of people with OCD and those with drug addiction, the cutting edge treatment for OCD might serve as a useful model when considering treatment for the neurobiochemical and neurophysiological aspects of addiction.

Neurobiochemistry in OCD

There are several known changes in neuronal signaling and neurobiochemistry that are characteristic to patients with OCD, compared to those without OCD or related mental disorders:

- alterations in serotonin synthesis, release, transport, sensitivity and metabolism; increasing synaptic levels of serotonin

- alterations in dopamine and noradrenaline synthesis, release, transport, sensitivity and metabolism

- alterations in glutamate and gamma-aminobutyric acid (GABA) synthesis, release, transport, sensitivity and metabolism.

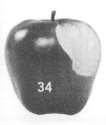

What can be inferred from current treatments used for OCD?

The main types of medical treatments used for OCD focus on increasing serotonergic signaling using selective serotonin reuptake inhibitors (SSRIs) and glutaminergic signaling using glutamate receptor agonists.

However, both serotonin production and signaling as well as glutamate production, transport and release are affected by diet and can be modulated by specific nutrients.

Serotonergic signaling and production can be enhanced by:

- supplementation with L-tryptophan or 5-hydroxy-tryptophan (these are serotonin precursors)
- vitamins B6, folate (vitamin B9) and vitamin B12 (important cofactors in the synthesis of serotonin)
- magnesium (an important cofactor in the synthesis of serotonin)
- omega-3 fatty acids (help to normalise serotonin sensitivity).

Glutamate production and release can be regulated by supplementation with:

- amino acid N-acetyl-cysteine (NAC), as cysteine plays an important role in the transport and release of glutamate at the appropriate time
- amino acid L-glutamine (a precursor to glutamate)
- vitamin B6 and magnesium (important cofactors in the enzyme that breaks down glutamate).

Dietary changes and nutritional interventions could therefore potentially also be used to manage the OCD-like aspects of addiction.

Oxidative stress

Increased cerebral oxidative stress seems to be part of the neurobiochemical problem in addiction. Numerous drugs and substances of abuse cause oxidative stress directly or indirectly.

- The excess glutamate released initially causes oxidative stress and eventually neuronal death.
- The excess release of dopamine can lead to states of oxidative stress as dopamine is easily oxidised, leading to the formation of neurotoxic

breakdown products that are toxic to dopaminergic cells and are very unstable, causing further oxidative stress.

- The generally unfavourable changes in diet resulting from drug abuse lead to an insufficient intake of antioxidants and phytochemicals that are either direct antioxidants or that stimulate the body's endogenous antioxidant defences.

- The smoking that usually accompanies addiction to harder drugs and stimulants than nicotine.

- The excess ingestion of alcohol that usually accompanies addiction to harder drugs and stimulants.

Oxidative stress plays a role in:

- the general decline in neuronal function and mental faculties seen with long-term drug abuse

- initiation of a stress response that subsequently increases the risk of relapse

- the changes in mood and emotions that cause the problems via changes in neurotransmitter production, release and transport.

Fortunately, a healthier diet, a healthier lifestyle and targeted nutritional supplementation can help lower oxidative stress systemically and cerebrally. See Box 2.1 for further information.

Box 2.1: Steps that can be taken to decrease oxidative stress

1. Eating at least 600g of vegetables, berries and fruits daily.

2. Eating crops that are specifically known to increase endogenous antioxidant capacity on a daily basis such as berries, vegetables of the Brassica family (broccoli, cabbage and radishes), vegetables of the Allium family (onions, spring onions, garlic, leeks and chives), turmeric, ginger, rosemary, thyme, oregano, sage, chili, green leafy vegetables and beets.

3. Eating whole grains instead of refined grains

4. Limiting the consumption of refined sugar to an absolute minimum

5. Eating moderate amounts of nuts and seeds

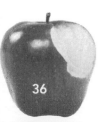

6.   Choosing high quality cold-pressed and unrefined vegetable oils rather than refined vegetable fats

7.   Eating game and organic, grass-fed animal products rather than products (meats, eggs, milk, yoghurt etc.) from feedlot raised, grain-fed animals

8.   Eating fish and seafood on a daily basis

9.   Drinking tea, green tea, white tea and vegetable juices

10. Exercising on a daily basis

11. Getting sufficient sleep

12. Lowering stress levels

13. Supplementing with nutrients and phytochemicals that support the body's endogenous antioxidant defence systems such as zinc, copper, manganese, selenium, vitamin B6, N-acetyl-cysteine, L-glutamine, resveratrol, green tea polyphenols, alpha-lipoic acid, vitamin B2, vitamin B3, and curcumin from turmeric

14. Supplementing with antioxidants such as vitamin C, vitamin E, alpha-lipoic acid, carotenoids, polyphenols from tea and berries, quercetin, and curcumin from turmeric

Summary of nutritional and lifestyle co-interventions

Given the available knowledge on the neurobiochemistry of addiction, and what we know about the influence of food, diet, nutritional status and lifestyle on neurobiochemistry, it is sensible to consider nutrition as a tool when treating and/or managing drug addiction.

Numerous practitioners such as orthomolecular doctors and psychiatrists, nutritional therapists, cutting edge dietitians and educational specialists have a large experience base, although clinical research in this area is urgently required.

Nutrition is not to be considered as a primary tool of treatment, but as a secondary intervention that will help increase the effect and success rate of primary, social and psychological interventions and treatments.

Why stabilise overall neurobiochemistry?

- Stabilise brain functioning and signaling, thus decreasing the triggers for wanting to abuse substances
- Normalise altered brain circuitry, neurotransmitter release and sensitivity following abuse
- Prevent the triggering of uncontrollable cravings
- Block or dampen the effects of stimulants

Suggested nutritional interventions

Glycaemic control

Controlling blood sugar levels is important for several reasons:

- rapid fluctuations in blood sugar levels can increase the production of stress hormones, and stress increases the risk of relapse
- fast increases in blood sugar levels may trigger the same responses and neuronal networks as substances of abuse, especially in susceptible individuals; this can increase the risk of relapse.

Blood sugar levels can be controlled by a combination of diet, exercise, supplementation and lifestyle changes.

- Avoid all refined sugars and other refined carbohydrates, and ingest modest amounts of fruits, whole grains, legumes and tubers instead
- Increase the intake of lean protein
- Ingest sufficient amounts of healthy fats
- Exercise daily, ideally ensuring that an exercise programme includes both endurance and strength training
- Ingest more fibre by increasing fibrous foods and possibly also taking supplements of fibre

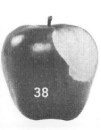

■ Increase the intake of vegetables, preferably berries rather than fruit, and preferably fresh fruit rather than dried fruit

■ Eat more regular but smaller meals

■ Get sufficient sleep as insufficient sleep is associated with poorer glycaemic control

■ Either avoid caffeine or only ingest moderate amounts as excess caffeine will destabilise blood sugar levels in some individuals

■ Decrease stress as the stress response can adversely affect blood sugar control

■ Magnesium, zinc, chromium and alpha-lipoic acid may help stabilise blood sugar levels

Omega-3 and omega-6 fatty acids

Essential fatty acids and their long-chain derivates eicosapentanoic acid (EPA), docosahexaenoic acid (DHA), arachidonic acid (AA) and di-homo-gamma-linolenic-acid (DGLA) all play important roles in brain functioning including:

■ modulating the synthesis, release, metabolism of dopamine, noradrenaline, serotonin and glutamate, and the sensitivity to them

■ increasing cerebral glutathione levels

■ blunting the release of stress hormones and decreasing cerebral sensitivity to the stress hormone cortisol.

> **Note:** The suggested dosage of EPA and DHA is in the range of 500mg to 10–15g per day either in triglyceride form or as ethyl-EPA.
> **Important:** Larger doses should only be consumed under medical supervision to prevent potential bleeding problems.

Folate, vitamins B6 and B12

Folate and vitamins B6 and B12 are respectively important co-factors in the synthesis and metabolism of one, several or all of the neurotransmitters affected by drugs (dopamine, noradrenaline, serotonin, glutamate, GABA) and that are altered in addiction. By increasing the availability of these three important co-factors, overall neurobiochemistry may be improved, helping to decrease neurobiochemical reactions and states that increase the urge to (re)use drugs.

Minerals and trace elements

Zinc, magnesium, copper and iron are all important co-factors in the sensitivity to, synthesis and metabolism of one or more of the neurotransmitters involved in addiction. Obtaining sufficient levels of these is important.

- A therapeutic dose of magnesium would be 300–1,000mg daily in an easily absorbable form such as magnesium citrate, magnesium asporotate or magnesium bisglycinate.

- A therapeutic dose of zinc would be 15–50mg daily in an easily absorbable form such as zinc citrate or zinc bisglycinate.

- A therapeutic dose of iron would be between 150µg and 1g daily, with higher dosages only to be used under supervision to avoid iron overload.

- A therapeutic dose of copper would be 2–4mg daily.

Calcium may also be necessary. Despite not being a co-factor in the synthesis or metabolism of any of the neurotransmitters affected in addiction, calcium is important for neurotransmission and insufficiencies could lead to altered neuronal functioning. It should be noted that calcium uptake and transport is only effective when sufficient vitamin D and vitamin K are ingested and/or present in the blood stream.

Finally, adequate selenium status should be considered. Selenium is an important co-factor in various antioxidant systems and overall brain health. Low selenium status or outright deficiency is often observed in addicts. A therapeutic dose of selenium would be 250–300 micrograms (mcg) daily.

N-acetyl-cysteine (NAC)

Providing supplements of the amino acid N-acetyl-cysteine (NAC) increases cerebral levels of the amino acids cysteine and cystine and has shown promise in the management of addiction because of its ability to optimise glutamate release and to protect against the damaging effects of excess glutamate.

Several small studies and trials with NAC supplementation in cocaine, cannabis and nicotine addiction, as well as in compulsive gambling and OCD, have shown promising effects. It should be noted that NAC was not solely responsible for treating these conditions. However, improvements in controlling the urge to engage in the unwanted behaviours and less abuse, gambling and compulsive actions were seen when NAC was supplemented. This could help increase the success rate of various rehabilitation programmes. The suggested dosage would be 600–2,400mg of NAC daily.

Inositol

Inositol is a carbohydrate that was previously classed as a B-vitamin. Inositol plays an important role as a secondary messenger in cell signaling, including responses to signals transmitted via serotonin, dopamine, noradrenalin, insulin and various other neurotransmitters, hormones and messaging systems.

Decreased levels of inositol have been observed in the cerebrospinal fluid of patients with various psychiatric conditions. A number of trials, including some blinded and placebo-controlled trials, have shown inositol to be efficacious in the management of depression, OCD and anxiety disorder. Considering the overlap of depression and anxiety with drug abuse as well as the similarities in OCD and drug addiction, supplementation of inositol as part of a broad approach to managing addiction may be relevant. The suggested dosage would be 12–18g daily.

Vitamin D

Vitamin D could also be considered in the nutritional management of addiction. Vitamin D is not only important for calcium absorption and bone density, but also has potent effects on the brain.

Vitamin D:

- stimulates neuroplasticity
- stimulates the release of brain-derived neurotrophic factor (BdNF), which is important for brain health and functioning
- has anti-inflammatory effects.

Impaired neuroplasticity, lower levels of BdNF and psychiatric disorders associated with increased cerebral inflammation are all issues in drug addiction – and these may be managed more effectively with sufficient vitamin D. The best way to ensure vitamin D adequacy is by taking a blood test. Optimal vitamin D levels are above 100 nmol/L (35ng/ml). If vitamin D levels are lower, supplementation or more exposure to sunshine should be considered.

Amino acids

Amino acids can help to support the synthesis of several of the neurotransmitters that are affected by addiction – normalisation of synthesis, transport and metabolism of these may be of benefit.

L-phenylalanine and L-tyrosine are precursors for dopamine and consequently also noradrenaline. Supplementation with either of these amino acids may help increase the production of dopamine and noradrenaline if required. Suggested doses are 500mg 1–3 times daily on an empty stomach, preferably starting upon rising. Furthermore, velvet bean concentrates or extracts contain L-dopa, which is the immediate precursor to dopamine.

L-tryptophan is the precursor for serotonin. Supplementation with L-tryptophan may help support serotonin synthesis, if required. Suggested doses are 500mg 1–3 times daily on an empty stomach.

Concentrates of or extracts from the seeds of Griffonia simplicifolia contain 5-hydroxytryptophan (5-HTP), which is the immediate precursor to serotonin. Suggested doses are 50–100mg of 5-HTP taken 1–3 times daily.

Note: Therapy with amino acids that are precursors to neurotransmitters should be closely supervised in patients who are taking prescribed medication affecting serotonin, dopamine and noradrenaline levels, as the addictive effects of both precursors and medications may lead to toxicity.

Other co-interventions

Meditation and mindfulness

Meditation and mindfulness work are likely to be of benefit in the management of neurobiochemical aspects of addiction. Both modalities affect numerous pathways, functions and biochemical reactions that can be manipulated to make it easier to break the cycle of addiction.

The specific effects are:

■ they increase neuroplasticity, which can make it easier to reverse the rewiring of neuronal circuitry that promotes addiction and dependence

■ they increase and modulate levels of dopamine, serotonin, glutamate and GABA; optimising and normalising levels of these neurotransmitters may be of benefit

■ they change the response to external inputs, including lowering the stress response to potentially noxious stimuli, decreasing the likelihood of relapse during stress

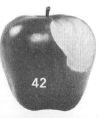

■ they lower the general stress response, also helping to decrease the likelihood of relapse during stress.

Exercise

Regular exercise also has beneficial effects on numerous targets in the management of the neurobiochemical aspects of addiction. Specifically:

■ the production of dopamine, serotonin, glutamate and GABA

■ reducing stress levels

■ improving neuroplasticity.

In order for these effects to be sufficiently strong to be of benefit, one has to exercise at moderate to high intensity for 30–60 minutes at least four times a week.

> **Note:** Nutritional supplementation is a highly specialised area and based on an individual's biochemical requirements. Expert medical advice should be sought before taking any high dose vitamin and mineral supplements, particularly if they are taken for an extended period of time.

Bibliography

Agudelo M, Gandhi N, Saiyed Z, Pichili V, Thangavel S, Khatavkar P, Yndart-Arias A & Nair M (2011) Effects of alcohol on histone deacetylase 2 (HDAC2) and the neuroprotective role of trichostatin A (TSA). *Alcoholism: Clinical and experimental research* **35** (8) 1550–1556.

Albert U, Bergesio C, Pessina E, Maina G & Bogetto F (2002) Management of treatment resistant obsessive-compulsive disorder. Algorithms for pharmacotherapy. *Panminerva Medica* **44** (2) 83–91.

Amen SL, Piacentine LB, Ahmad ME, Li SJ, Mantsch JR, Risinger RC & Baker DA (2011) Repeated N-acetyl cysteine reduces cocaine seeking in rodents and craving in cocaine-dependent humans. *Neuropsychopharmacology* **36** (4) 871–878.

Bedard MJ & Chantal S (2011) Brain magnetic resonance spectroscopy in obsessive-compulsive disorder: the importance of considering subclinical symptoms of anxiety and depression. *Psychiatry Research* **192** (1) 45–54.

Berk M, Jeavons S, Dean OM, Dodd S, Moss K, Gama CS & Malhi GS (2009) Nail-biting stuff? The effect of N-acetyl cysteine on nail-biting. *CNS Spectrums* **14** (7) 357-360.

Bersudsky Y, Einat H, Stahl Z & Belmaker RH (1999) Epi-inositol and inositol depletion: two new treatment approaches in affective disorder. *Current Psychiatry Reports* **1** (2) 141–147.

Brink CB, Viljoen SL, de Kock SE, Stein DJ & Harvey BH (2004) Effects of myo-inositol versus fluoxetine and imipramine pretreatments on serotonin 5HT2A and muscarinic acetylcholine receptors in human neuroblastoma cells. *Metabolic Brain Disease* **19** (1–2) 51–70.

Camfield DA, Sarris J & Berk M (2011) Nutraceuticals in the treatment of obsessive compulsive disorder (OCD): a review of mechanistic and clinical evidence. *Progress in Neuropsychopharmacology & Biological Psychiatry* **35** (4) 887–895.

Carvalho F (2009) How bad is accelerated senescence in consumers of drugs of abuse? *Adicciones* **21** (2) 99–104.

Chinta SJ & Andersen JK (2005) Dopaminergic neurons. *International Journal of Biochemistry and Cell Biology* **37** (5) 942–946.

Colodny L & Hoffman RL (1998) Inositol – clinical applications for exogenous use. *Alternative Medicine Review* **3** (6) 432–447.

Cui J, Shao L, Young LT & Wang JF (2007) Role of glutathione in neuroprotective effects of mood stabilizing drugs lithium and valproate. *Neuroscience* **144** (4) 1447–1453.

Cunha-Oliveira T, Rego AC & Oliveira CR (2008) Cellular and molecular mechanisms involved in the neurotoxicity of opioid and psychostimulant drugs. *Brain Research Reviews* **58** (1) 192–208.

Dean O, Giorlando F & Berk M (2011) N-acetylcysteine in psychiatry: current therapeutic evidence and potential mechanisms of action. *Journal of Psychiatry & Neuroscience* **36** (2) 78–86.

Einat H & Belmaker RH (2001) The effects of inositol treatment in animal models of psychiatric disorders. *Journal of Affective Disorders* **62** (1–2) 113–121.

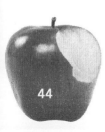

Freeman MP, Freeman SA & McElroy SL (2002) The comorbidity of bipolar and anxiety disorders: prevalence, psychobiology, and treatment issues. *Journal of Affective Disorders* **68** (1) 1–23.

Fux M, Benjamin J & Belmaker RH (1999) Inositol versus placebo augmentation of serotonin reuptake inhibitors in the treatment of obsessive-compulsive disorder: a double-blind cross-over study. *International Journal of Neuropsychopharmacology* **2** (3) 193–195.

Fux M, Levine J, Aviv A & Belmaker RH (1996) Inositol treatment of obsessive-compulsive disorder. *American Journal of Psychiatry* **153** (9) 1219–1221.

Gass JT & Olive MF (2008) Glutamatergic substrates of drug addiction and alcoholism. *Biochemical Pharmacology* **75** (1) 218–265.

Grant JE, Kim SW & Odlaug BL (2007) N-acetyl cysteine, a glutamate-modulating agent, in the treatment of pathological gambling: a pilot study. *Biological Psychiatry* **62** (6) 652–657.

Gray KM, Watson NL, Carpenter MJ & Larowe SD (2010) N-acetylcysteine (NAC) in young marijuana users: an open-label pilot study. American *Journal on Addictions* **19** (2) 187–189.

Harvey BH, Brink CB, Seedat S & Stein DJ (2002) Defining the neuromolecular action of myo-inositol: application to obsessive-compulsive disorder. *Progress in Neuropsychopharmacology & Biological Psychiatry* **26** (1) 21–32.

Jorm AF, Christensen H, Griffiths KM, Parslow RA, Rodgers B & Blewitt KA (2004) Effectiveness of complementary and self-help treatments for anxiety disorders. *Medical Journal of Australia* **181** (7) 29–46.

Karila L, Gorelick D, Weinstein A, Noble F, Benyamina A, Coscas S, Blecha L, Lowenstein W, Martinot JL, Reynaud M & Lépine JP (2008) New treatments for cocaine dependence: a focused review. *International Journal of Neuropsychopharmacology* **11** (3) 425–438.

Karila L & Reynaud M (2009) Therapeutic approaches to cocaine addiction. *La Revue du Practicien* **59** (6) 830–834.

Karila L, Weinstein A, Benyamina A, Coscas S, Leroy C, Noble F, Lowenstein W, Aubin HJ, Lépine JP & Reynaud M (2008) Current pharmacotherapies and immunotherapy in cocaine addiction. *Presse Medicale* **37** (2) 689–698.

Kim H, McGrath BM & Silverstone PH (2005) A review of the possible relevance of inositol and the phosphatidylinositol second messenger system (PI-cycle) to psychiatric disorders–focus on magnetic resonance spectroscopy (MRS) studies. *Human Psychopharmacology* **20** (5) 309–326.

Kinrys G, Coleman E & Rothstein E (2009) Natural remedies for anxiety disorders: potential use and clinical applications. *Depression & Anxiety* **26** (3) 259–265.

Kovacic P (2005) Role of oxidative metabolites of cocaine in toxicity and addiction: oxidative stress and electron transfer. *Medical Hypotheses* **64** (2) 350–356.

Kovacic P (2005) Unifying mechanism for addiction and toxicity of abused drugs with application to dopamine and glutamate mediators: electron transfer and reactive oxygen species. *Medical Hypotheses* **65** (1) 90–96.

Kovacic P & Cooksy AL (2005) Unifying mechanism for toxicity and addiction by abused drugs: electron transfer and reactive oxygen species. *Medical Hypotheses* **64** (2) 357–366.

Lai JS, Zhao C, Warsh JJ & Li PP (2006) Cytoprotection by lithium and valproate varies between cell types and cellular stresses. *European Journal of Pharmacology* **539** (1–2) 18–26.

LaRowe SD, Myrick H, Hedden S, Mardikian P, Saladin M, McRae A, Brady K, Kalivas PW & Malcolm R (2007) Is cocaine desire reduced by N-acetylcysteine? *American Journal of Psychiatry* **164** (7) 1115–1117.

Levine J (1997) Controlled trials of inositol in psychiatry. *European Neuropsychopharmacology* **7** (2) 147–155.

Madayag A, Kau KS, Lobner D, Mantsch JR, Wisniewski S & Baker DA (2010) Drug-induced plasticity contributing to heightened relapse susceptibility: neurochemical changes and augmented reinstatement in high-intake rats. *Journal of Neuroscience* **30** (1) 210–217.

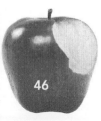

Madayag A, Lobner D, Kau KS, Mantsch JR, Abdulhameed O, Hearing M, Grier MD & Baker DA (2007) Repeated N-acetylcysteine administration alters plasticity-dependent effects of cocaine. *Journal of Neuroscience* **27** (51) 13968–13976.

Mirecki A, Fitzmaurice P, Ang L, Kalasinsky KS, Peretti FJ, Aiken SS, Wickham DJ, Sherwin A, Nobrega JN, Forman HJ & Kish SJ (2004) Brain antioxidant systems in human methamphetamine users. *Journal of Neurochemistry* **8** (6) 1396–1408.

Moussawi K, Pacchioni A, Moran M, Olive MF, Gass JT, Lavin A & Kalivas PW (2009) N-Acetylcysteine reverses cocaine-induced metaplasticity. *Nature Neuroscience* **12** (2) 182–189.

Moussawi K, Zhou W, Shen H, Reichel CM, See RE, Carr DB & Kalivas PW (2011) Reversing cocaine-induced synaptic potentiation provides enduring protection from relapse. *Proceedings of the National Academy of Sciences USA* **108** (1) 385–390.

Muriach M, López-Pedrajas R, Barcia JM, Sanchez-Villarejo MV, Almansa I & Romero FJ (2010) Cocaine causes memory and learning impairments in rats: involvement of nuclear factor kappa B and oxidative stress, and prevention by topiramate. *Journal of Neurochemistry* **114** (3) 675–684.

Nemets B, Fux M, Levine J & Belmaker RH (2001) Combination of antidepressant drugs: the case of inositol. *Human Psychopharmacology* **16** (1) 37–43.

Palatnik A, Frolov K, Fux M & Benjamin J (2001) Double-blind, controlled, crossover trial of inositol versus fluvoxamine for the treatment of panic disorder. *Journal of Clinical Psychopharmacology* **21** (3) 335–339.

Patel J, Manjappa N, Bhat R, Mehrotra P, Bhaskaran M & Singhal PC (2003) Role of oxidative stress and heme oxygenase activity in morphine-induced glomerular epithelial cell growth. *American Journal of Physiology. Renal Physiology* **285** (5) 861–869.

Patkar AA, Rozen S, Mannelli P, Matson W, Pae CU, Krishnan KR & Kaddurah-Daouk R (2009) Alterations in tryptophan and purine metabolism in cocaine addiction: a metabolomic study. *Psychopharmacology (Berl)* **206** (3) 479–489.

Pereska Z, Dejanova B, Bozinovska C & Petkovska L (2007) Prooxidative/antioxidative homeostasis in heroin addiction and detoxification. *Bratislava Medical Journal* **108** (9) 393–398.

Poon HF, Abdullah L, Mullan MA, Mullan MJ & Crawford FC (2007) Cocaine-induced oxidative stress precedes cell death in human neuronal progenitor cells. *Neurochemistry International* **50** (1) 69–73.

Rosenberg DR, Mirza Y, Russell A, Tang J, Smith JM, Banerjee SP, Bhandari R, Rose M, Ivey J, Boyd C & Moore GJ (2004) Reduced anterior cingulate glutamatergic concentrations in childhood OCD and major depression versus healthy controls. *Journal of the American Academy of Child and Adolescent Psychiatry* **43** (9) 1146–1153.

Saeed SA, Bloch RM & Antonacci DJ (2007) Herbal and dietary supplements for treatment of anxiety disorders. *American Family Physician* **76** (4) 549–556.

Sarris J, Camfield D & Berk M (2011) Complementary medicine, self-help, and lifestyle interventions for obsessive compulsive disorder (OCD) and the OCD spectrum: a systematic review. *Journal of Affective Disorders* May 25 [Epub ahead of print].

Seedat S & Stein DJ (1999) Inositol augmentation of serotonin reuptake inhibitors in treatment-refractory obsessive-compulsive disorder: an open trial. *International & Clinical Psychopharmacology* **14** (6) 353–356.

Seedat S, Stein DJ & Harvey BH (2001) Inositol in the treatment of trichotillomania and compulsive skin picking. *Journal of Clinical Psychiatry* **62** (1) 60–61.

Shiba T, Yamato M, Kudo W, Watanabe T, Utsumi H & Yamada K (2011) In vivo imaging of mitochondrial function in methamphetamine-treated rats. *Neuroimage* **57** (3) 866–872.

Silva AP, Martins T, Baptista S, Gonçalves J, Agasse F & Malva JO (2010) Brain injury associated with widely abused amphetamines: neuroinflammation, neurogenesis and blood-brain barrier. *Current Drug Abuse Reviews* **3** (4) 239–254.

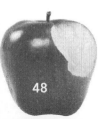

Tata DA & Yamamoto BK (2007) Interactions between methamphetamine and environmental stress: role of oxidative stress, glutamate and mitochondrial dysfunction. *Addiction* **102** (1) 49–60.

Uys JD & LaLumiere RT (2008) Glutamate: the new frontier in pharmacotherapy for cocaine addiction. *CNS & Neurological Disorders Drug Targets* **7** (5) 482–491.

Yücel M, Wood SJ, Wellard RM, Harrison BJ, Fornito A, Pujol J, Velakoulis D & Pantelis C (2008) Anterior cingulate glutamate-glutamine levels predict symptom severity in women with obsessive-compulsive disorder. *Australian & New Zealand Journal of Psychiatry* **42** (6) 467–477.

Zhou W (2010) Normalizing drug-induced neuronal plasticity in nucleus accumbens weakens enduring drug-seeking behavior. *Neuropsychopharmacology* **35** (1) 352–353.

Further reading

Bland J & Jones D (2005) Clinical approaches to hormonal and neuroendocrine imbalances – cellular messaging, part 1. In: D Jones & S Quinn (Eds) *The Textbook of Functional Medicine*. Gig Harbor, WA: The Institute For Functional Medicine.

Hyman M (2009) *The UltraMind Solution*. New York: Scribner.

Liska D (2005) Influence of mind and spirit. In: D Jones & S Quinn (Eds) *The Textbook of Functional Medicine*. Gig Harbor, WA: The Institute For Functional Medicine.

Hedaya R, Quinn S & Jones D (2008) *Depression: Advancing the treatment paradigm (functional medicine clinical monographs)*. Gig Harbor, WA: The Institute For Functional Medicine.

Hedaya R (1996) *Understanding Biological Psychiatry*. New York: WW Norton.

Hedaya R (2001) *The Antidepressant Survival Guide: The clinically proven program to enhance the benefits and beat the side effects of your medication*. California: Three Rivers Press.

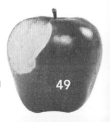

Lombard J (2005) Clinical approaches to hormonal and neuroendocrine imbalances – neurotransmitters: A functional medicine approach to neuropsychiatry. In: D Jones & S Quinn (Eds) *The Textbook of Functional Medicine*. Gig Harbor, WA: The Institute For Functional Medicine.

Ross J (2003) *The Mood Cure: The 4-Step change program to take charge of your emotions today*. Penguin Group USA: Penguin.

Willner C (2005) Neurological imbalances. In: D Jones & S Quinn (Eds) *The Textbook of Functional Medicine*. Gig Harbor, WA: The Institute for Functional Medicine.

Chapter 3

Diet in substance misusers and the prison population

Helen Sandwell

Introduction

Substance use involves the consumption of alcohol, drugs or other chemicals such as solvents, which are often psychoactive or performance-enhancing in their action. For most, substance use takes place at a level which is acceptable and legitimate within society, for example 'sensible' drinking or cigarette smoking. When harm is caused to the individual involved (or those around them) as a result of taking the substance, this activity is no longer seen as a socially acceptable pastime and is termed 'substance misuse' or 'problem substance use'.

Dependency or addiction occurs when substance misuse becomes compulsive and repetitive. Dependency may result in tolerance to the effect of the drug and increasingly greater amounts are needed to be taken to achieve the desired effect. For those dependent on a substance, psychological and/or physiological withdrawal symptoms can occur when use is reduced or stopped. In some instances, such as with heavy alcohol dependency, physiological withdrawal can be so severe that it becomes life-threatening and withdrawal must take place under medical supervision.

Substance misuse is rarely the sole negative influence on an individual's life. It is often just one aspect of a complex array of detrimental factors, which all interact with each other and compound an individual's problems.[1] These factors may also include poverty; weak family support structure or family breakdown; childhood neglect or abuse; domestic violence; growing up in a

---

1   Rankin J & Regan S (2004) *Meeting Complex Needs: The future of social care*. London: Institute for Public Policy Research & Turning Point.

family where parental substance misuse hampers parenting; learning and behavioural difficulties; mental health problems; lack of education, training and employment opportunities; underachievement; poor diet; and overall low resilience. In the same way, improving diet is just one small but important part of the jigsaw that can contribute to building resilience and can help individuals abstain from or minimise harm from drugs and alcohol.

Eating a balanced diet – when also combined with increasing knowledge around food shopping, cooking and a positive attitude towards the social aspects of eating – can help individuals to build a rewarding life beyond substance misuse. Improving the diets of drug and alcohol users should always be viewed in a far wider context than encouraging them to take a nutrient supplement. This chapter focuses on issues around diet and physical and mental health that are specific to people with drug and alcohol dependencies. It also looks at the personal circumstances that can act as barriers to people making healthy food choices and how a balanced diet, together with other lifestyle factors, can support an individual through drug and alcohol treatment.

Nutritional status of drug and alcohol users

It is obvious to those who work with people who have drug or alcohol dependencies that their clients have poor eating habits and are likely to have nutrient deficiencies. Such observations are supported by research studies looking at the diets and nutritional status of substance misusers. For example, several deficiencies have been identified among drug users, including the deficiency of vitamin A, B6, C and E and folic acid.[2,3] Notably, folic acid is a key nutrient associated with mood and mental health, and needs vitamin B6 to work effectively. Vitamins A, C and E are antioxidants which, among other functions, are important for fighting infections. Poor mental health and infections are both common health risks for substance misusers and are compounded by dietary deficiencies.

2   El Nakah A (1979) A vitamin profile of heroin addiction. *American Journal of Public Health* **69** (10) 1058–1060.

3   Nazrul Islam SK, Jahangir Hossain K & Ahsan M (2001) Serum vitamin E, C and A status of the drug addicts undergoing detoxification: influence of drug habit, sexual practice and lifestyle factors. *European Journal of Clinical Nutrition* **55** (11) 1022–1027.

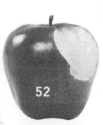

Thiamin (vitamin B1) deficiency is common in heavy drinkers as a result of inadequate intake, decreased absorption in the gut and impaired utilisation by cells. This can lead to Wernicke's encephalopathy typified by jerky abnormal eye movements, loss of muscle co-ordination and a confused state. Orally or intravenously administered thiamin is used to reverse the effects of deficiency. However, in the later stages, irreversible brain damage may occur, known as Korsakoff's psychosis, which is characterised by severe memory problems. Together these conditions are commonly known as Wernicke-Korsakoff syndrome.

Eating patterns and dietary choices are often severely affected during periods of substance misuse. See Box 3.1. Meals will frequently be missed altogether and food that is consumed is likely to be whatever can be eaten quickly and easily. For heavy drinkers, the alcohol damage to the intestinal tract may make eating anything more than a small portion of the plainest food very difficult.

Box 3.1: Quotes from service users

'I live on chocolate and ice cream when I take drugs. I eat chocolate for a quick fix'.

'I can go six days without eating anything.'

(Participants in a prison drug treatment programme in a high security prison)

Poor food choices are common. Vegetable consumption has been shown to be significantly lower for drug users and the consumption of sweets or desserts significantly higher compared to non-drug user controls.[4] In Himmelgreen's (1998) study of the nutritional status and food security of drug-using and non-drug-using Hispanic women in Hartford, Connecticut, drug users were more likely to fry food, whereas controls were more likely to bake, boil or steam.

Malnutrition can adversely affect a person's mood, sleep patterns and concentration. A study of 22 undernourished patients (weight loss>5% in one month or BMI<20) showed that tension, depression, anger, vigour, fatigue and confusion all improved significantly following eight days of nutrition treatment.[5] It is no wonder then that poor nutrition could further worsen negative mood and behaviour in substance misusers who may well already have an underlying mood disorder, which is exacerbated by the effects of drugs or alcohol.

---

4   Himmelgreen D (1998) A comparison of the nutritional status and food security of drug-using and non-drug-using Hispanic women in Hartford, Connecticut. *American Journal of Physical Anthropology* **107** (3) 351–361.

5   Stanga Z (2007) The effect of nutritional management on the mood of malnourished patients. *Clinical Nutrition* **26** 379–382.

The disordered eating often associated with substance misuse may be only one step away from an eating disorder. Eating disorders and substance misuse, particularly the use of appetite suppressing stimulant drugs, are common comorbidities, predominantly in women. An estimated 50% of people with eating disorders also have drug or alcohol problems.[6] It is also thought that chronic dietary restriction can enhance the drug reward mechanism[7], so undereating may be used by some, albeit subconsciously, to help increase a drug high. It can be difficult to differentiate between what came first – the eating disorder or the drug dependency – as they may well be symptoms with a common root cause.

Personal circumstances affecting diet

As well as the specific effects of the drugs on food intake and nutrient status, there are many factors common to the lives of those with drug or alcohol dependency, which can further contribute to poor food choices and a poor diet.

Lack of money, or money preferentially being used for drugs, is an overriding factor contributing to poor diet. The strong psychological and/or physiological need for drugs in someone with a dependency is likely to prevent them from spending their often limited resources on food.

Box 3.2: Quote from a service user

'When you're sick [in withdrawal] you can't eat, and when you're stoned you don't care if you're hungry, but you can't afford to eat anyway.'

(A service user/trainer, Council for the Homeless, Northern Ireland)

A lack of knowledge around healthy eating and cooking as well as poor literacy and numeracy skills can also contribute to making poor food choices. The *FAB! Food and Wellbeing programme* – a healthy eating programme run by Food Matters for vulnerable adults, many of whom are substance misusers – has found that many of the participants had left school at 16 or younger, with few or no qualifications, had never worked and had little experience of cooking.

---

6   CASA (The National Center on Addiction and Substance Abuse at Columbia University) (2001) *CASA Conference: Food for Thought – Substance abuse and eating disorders*. New York: Columbia University.

7   Cabeza de Vaca S & Karr AD (1998) Food restriction enhances the central rewarding effect of abused drugs. *Journal of Neuroscience* **18** (18) 7502–7510.

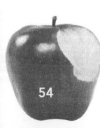

For many substance misusers living arrangements can compromise their food choices. Those who are homeless and living on the street are dependent on pre-prepared food, either from soup kitchens, shops or catering establishments and often, fast food outlets. At the time of writing there are still people living on the streets with drug or alcohol dependencies who have no means of income and are completely reliant on food provided by not-for-profit organisations. For them, the healthiness of a meal is not their top priority, but whether they have access to food at all.

For the homeless dependent on 'crash pad' emergency hostels and 'sofa surfers' who rely on the generosity of friends to provide a temporary place to sleep, the lack of a permanent base means they do not have the opportunity to shop, stock a food cupboard or cook. Without secure homes of their own, and without cooking and food storage facilities, individuals can feel they have little control over their food choices.

Diet related health concerns

People with a history of substance misuse are likely to have adverse health outcomes relating to their drug or alcohol dependency. Since poly-drug use is common among substance misusers, related health problems can be multiple and complex. Often these health concerns can be worsened by poor diet. On the upside, improving diet can help improve physical health and can help slow the progression of some chronic illnesses.

Alcohol

As previously mentioned, Wernicke-Korsakoff syndrome, a condition that is commonly seen in street drinkers with prolonged histories of heavy drinking, is caused by thiamin deficiency. Brain damage can develop, which is further compounded by the direct toxic effects of alcohol on the brain.

Liver damage is also a major concern for heavy drinkers. A certain amount of liver damage is reversible, with abstention from alcohol, but ongoing sustained heavy drinking can result in an inflamed hepatic liver that can become scarred and irreparably damaged (cirrhosis). A poor diet can also be detrimental to liver health so it is important for anyone with liver damage to eat a nutritious, balanced diet to help maintain overall health and to help slow the rate of liver damage.

Additionally, damage to the pancreas and gut lining are common in heavy drinkers. Overall, these can seriously affect the body's ability to absorb and process nutrients, in turn contributing to a state of poor nutrition and subsequent detrimental effects on health. Pancreatic damage can result in reduced levels of digestive enzymes being produced. Insulin production may also be disrupted, which may ultimately lead to the development of diabetes.

Injecting drugs

Liver damage can also result from certain viral infections. Among injecting drug users (IDUs) the most commonly seen blood-borne viral infection is hepatitis C, which is often passed on through the sharing of needles and other injecting paraphernalia. This often silent disease may go unnoticed for many years, with liver damage progressing undetected until symptoms of more advanced liver disease, cirrhosis and liver cancer become apparent. The Health Protection Agency's *Shooting Up* report stated that *'approaching one in two IDUs in the UK have been infected with hepatitis C',*[7] although not all will go on to develop advanced liver disease, and around 25% of those infected will spontaneously clear the virus completely.[8]

Nutritional status certainly impacts on the progression of the disease and specific nutrients are important for immunity, fighting infection and combating oxidative stress. Notably, low levels of plasma selenium are a risk factor for developing liver cancer among individuals with hepatitis B and C.[9] Like other liver diseases, muscle wasting is a common feature due to the liver's reduced capability to process protein. Small, frequent, protein-containing meals through the day are thought to be the most efficient way of the body being able to utilise dietary protein in this instance.

7 Health Protection Agency (2006) *Shooting Up: Infections among injecting drug users in the United Kingdom 2005. An update: October 2006.* London: HPA.

8   Micallef JM, Kaldor JM & Dore GJ (2006) Spontaneous viral clearance following acute hepatitis C infection: a systematic review of longitudinal studies. *Journal of Viral Hepatitis* **13** 34–41.

9   Yu M, Horng IS, Hsu KH, Chiang YC, Liaw YF & Chen CJ (1999) Selenium levels and risk of hepatocellular carcinoma among men with chronic hepatitis virus infection plasma. *American Journal of Epidemiology* **150** 367–374.

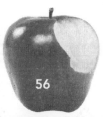

Important

Drug and alcohol users showing signs of advanced liver disease (ascites, varices, encephalopathy jaundice) should always be referred to a dietician for more specialised advice on eating, as should someone of low body weight who has lost weight unintentionally, anyone who has difficulty eating and swallowing, and anyone who requires dietary advice for an accompanying medical condition.

IDUs are susceptible to many other types of infection as a result of sharing equipment, using dirty equipment and through risky injecting methods. Bacterial infections can give rise to a heart (endocarditis) or bone (osteomyelitis) infection and abscesses. Poor diet, malnutrition and nutrient deficiencies reduce the body's resistance to infection, resulting in poor wound healing and persistent infections. Specific nutrients are known to be important for immunity and fighting infection (see Table 3.1).

Table 3.1: Dietary sources of some important nutrients associated with immune function

Nutrient	Dietary sources of nutrient
Vitamin A	Cheese, eggs, oily fish, liver, milk, fortified vegetable oil spreads and dried milk
Vitamin C	Fruit and vegetables, particularly citrus fruits
Vitamin D	Liver, oily fish, eggs, milk, fortified breakfast cereal, fortified vegetable oil spreads and dried milk; sunlight
Vitamin K	Green leafy vegetables, vegetable oils, cereals
Zinc	Meat, dairy, seafood and cereals
Selenium	Brazil nuts, eggs, offal, meat, fish, seafood
Iron	Red meat, liver, nuts, beans, wholegrains, dark green leafy vegetables, bread, fortified breakfast cereals

However, taking nutritional supplements, particularly single nutrient supplements, is rarely the best way to achieve an overall balanced diet. Single nutrient supplements can have negative effects, for example taking folic acid without vitamins B6 and B12 can mask the effects of vitamin B12 deficiency. A single multi-vitamin and mineral supplement is a safer option. There are times when specific nutrient supplements are helpful, for example when nutrient deficiencies are diagnosed, but it is always advisable to consult a dietician or doctor before doing this. Rather than targeting specific nutrients, the long-term aim should be to achieve an overall balanced diet containing sufficient levels of all nutrients, such as represented by the Eatwell Plate (Figure 3.1).

Figure 3.1: Eatwell Plate

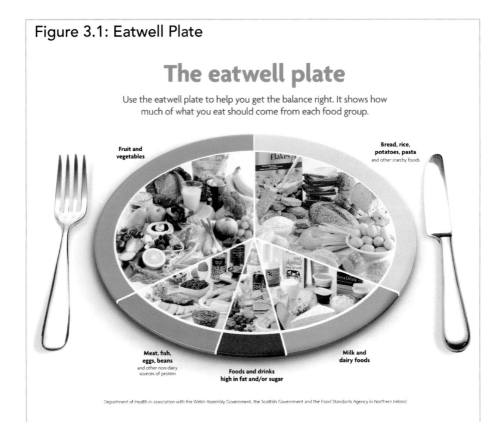

Reproduced with permission from the Department of Health in association with the Welsh Assembly Government, the Scottish Government and the Food Standards Agency in Northern Ireland. © Crown Copyright

The Eatwell Plate shows how much of what you eat should from each food group. This includes everything you eat during the day, including snacks.

So, try to eat:

- plenty of fruit and vegetables
- plenty of bread, rice, potatoes, pasta and other starchy foods – choose wholegrain varieties whenever you can
- some milk and dairy foods
- some meat, fish, eggs, beans and other non-dairy sources of protein
- just a small amount of foods and drinks high in fat and/or sugar.

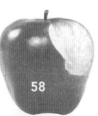

Oral health

Oral health refers to the health of the mouth, including soft tissue such as gums and teeth, and is often an area of concern for drug and alcohol users. Poor oral health is widespread among those with a drug or alcohol dependency. A survey of 220 methadone users in Dublin found 99% of subjects needed some form of dental treatment and the average number of teeth needing intervention was 14.[10] However, it is unlikely that it is simply the sugariness of methodone linctus that causes decay, as many think, since the same study found no greater rate of decay among individuals taking methadone sweetened with sugar compared to those taking methadone sweetened with an artificial sweetener. The decay process is likely to have started long before individuals began methadone treatment.

Table 3.2: Factors contributing to poor oral health in drug and alcohol users

- Years of neglect with poor oral hygiene
- Not visiting a dentist
- Individuals being unable to access NHS dental treatment or being refused dental treatment
- Poor diet and nutrient deficiencies
- High sugar intakes among some drug and alcohol users
- The xerostomic (dry mouth) effect of opiates promotes bacterial growth
- Damage to the tooth enamel from stomach acid through vomiting and from excessive carbonated drinks
- Tooth loss and damage through trauma, at times of inebriation
- Jaw clenching with stimulant use resulting in cracks in teeth
- Grinding teeth (bruxism) especially with stimulant use
- Smoking leading to increased risk of periodontal disease and mouth/throat cancer

---

Neglect of dental hygiene is just one of the factors contributing to poor oral health. Table 3.2 lists other factors. Poor diet and vitamin deficiencies can be the cause of mouth sores, fissures in the tongue and may weaken the jaw bone. In turn, poor oral health has a detrimental effect on diet by negatively impacting on food choices. If tooth loss, decay or soreness and inflammation in the mouth means that eating certain foods is difficult or

---

10   Gray R (2005) The oral effects of methadone use. *Network* (Substance Misuse Management in General Practice) **10** 1–3.

painful, it is likely that these foods will be avoided. Fruit and vegetables, particularly if raw and crunchy, are generally avoided among people who have considerable tooth loss. Softer, easier to eat foods, such as cakes and other sugary, fatty foods may replace them, thus contributing to the 'poor diet–poor oral health' cycle. Professionals who work with people who have severe tooth loss can help by advising them on softer fruit and vegetable alternatives, such as mashed and cooked fruit and vegetables, pureed vegetable soups and fruit smoothies.

Cycles of poor health

Like others caught in the poverty trap, another vicious cycle of '*poverty-poor diet-poor physical and mental health and impaired cognitive functioning*'[11] can be set up (See Figure 3.2). This can be further worsened when physical health is also compromised by substance misuse. This cycle can pass on down the generations when poor maternal diet impacts on foetal development. Damage to foetal development is further compounded by maternal alcohol or drug use.

Iron deficiency anaemia has been found to be extremely high in female inner city injecting drug users with HIV and/or hepatitis C infections.[12] This single nutrient deficiency alone can have a big effect on the capacity to learn, work and cope with day-to-day demands, since deficiency leads to reduced energy, lower aerobic capacity, decreased endurance and fatigue. It is thought that this in turn helps perpetuate the cycle of poverty by reducing work output and women's ability to remain in a job, education and training (Figure 3.3).

11   Vorster HH & Gibney MJ (2009) Food and nutrition-related diseases: the global challenge. In: Gibney MJ, Lanham-New SA, Cassidy A &Vorster HH (Eds) *Introduction to Human Nutrition* (2nd edition). Chichester: Wiley-Blackwell.

12   Semba D (2003) Iron-deficiency anemia and the cycle of poverty among human immunodeficiency virus-infected women in the inner city. *Clinical Infectious Diseases* **37** (2) 105–111.

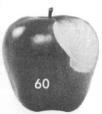

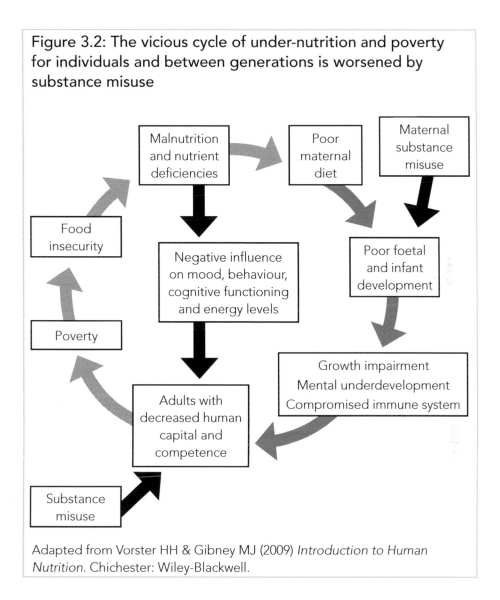

Figure 3.2: The vicious cycle of under-nutrition and poverty for individuals and between generations is worsened by substance misuse

Adapted from Vorster HH & Gibney MJ (2009) *Introduction to Human Nutrition*. Chichester: Wiley-Blackwell.

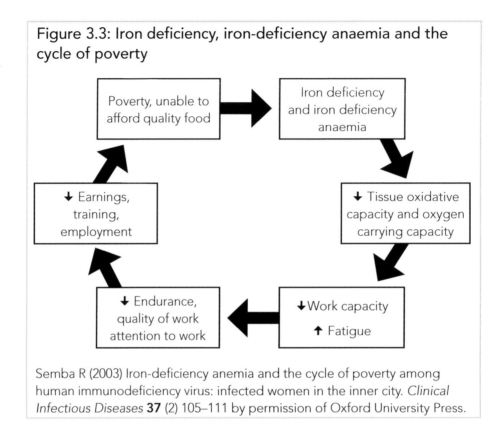

Figure 3.3: Iron deficiency, iron-deficiency anaemia and the cycle of poverty

Semba R (2003) Iron-deficiency anemia and the cycle of poverty among human immunodeficiency virus: infected women in the inner city. *Clinical Infectious Diseases* **37** (2) 105–111 by permission of Oxford University Press.

Diet, mood and behaviour in drug and alcohol users

Despite the mounting research on the relationship between food and mood, surprisingly little research has focused on diet relating to the mood and behaviour of those who misuse substances. This is surprising as people who misuse drugs or alcohol often have an underlying mood disorder and use drugs and alcohol as a means of self-medication. At the same time this group has probably among the poorest diets in our society. Negative mood can also be compounded by the effects of the drugs or withdrawal from them and by the physical ill-health often accompanying substance misuse. Overall, this group would appear to be among those who could benefit greatly from the potential links between improved diet and improved mood and behaviour. However, since substance misuse is still often seen by a large part of society as a problem caused by individuals themselves, such research involving this group is less likely to attract much funding. This is also a difficult group to study, since the risk of relapse and other possible factors, such as the chaotic behaviours and underlying mood disorders of many people in treatment, are likely to contribute to rates of non-compliance and the difficulties of conducting research in this group.

Nutrients and mood

Nonetheless, research in other subject groups relating to diet, mood and behaviour is accumulating. One major area of study has been that of the omega-3 polyunsaturated fatty acids (PUFAs), specifically eicosapentaenoic acid (EPA) and docosahexaenoic acid (DHA), which are found in substantial quantities in oily fish and fish oil. A meta-analysis of pooled data from 35 studies found that although there was a lack of evidence about the positive effect of omega-3 PUFAs on lesser states of depressed mood, the data suggested that omega-3 supplementation could positively affect major clinical depression.[13] Another meta-analysis, which looked at the effect of omega-3 in treating a range of psychiatric disorders, found that there was a significant benefit for the treatment of major and bipolar depression, though less benefit for schizophrenia.[14] A more recent systematic review looked at the effect of omega-3 on bipolar disorder alone.[15] Although only a small number of studies met their rigorous criteria for inclusion, and only one of these provided data for analysis, it suggested that as an adjunct, omega-3 could relieve the depressive but not the manic symptoms of bipolar disorder.

Other nutrients studied in relation to mood include folic acid and zinc. A study of 2,313 Finnish depressive patients who were followed for over 10 years showed that those with lower levels of folic acid were more likely to be diagnosed with depression again, compared to those with higher levels of folic acid.[16] Intervention studies have focused on using folic acid alongside standard medication. A meta-analysis of three double-blind placebo-controlled studies concluded that folic acid may have a potential

13   Appleton KM, Rogers PJ & Ness AR (2010) Updated systematic review and meta-analysis of the effects of n-3 long-chain polyunsaturated fatty acids on depressed mood. *American Journal of Clinical Nutrition* **91** (3) 757–770.

14   Freeman MP, Hibbeln JR, Wisner KL, Davis JM, Mischoulon D, Peet M, Keck PE Jr, Marangell LB, Richardson AJ, Lake J & Stoll AL (2006) Omega-3 fatty acids: evidence base for treatment and future research in psychiatry. *Journal of Clinical Psychiatry* **67** 1954–1967.

15   Montgomery P & Richardson AJ (2008) Omega-3 fatty acids for bipolar disorder. *Cochrane Database of Systematic Reviews* **2** CD005169.

16   Tolmunen T, Hintikka J, Ruusunen A, Voutilainen S, Tanskanen A, Valkonen VP, Viinamäki H, Kaplan GA & Salonen JT (2004) Dietary folate and the risk of depression in Finnish middle-aged men: a prospective follow-up study. *Psychotherapy and Psychosomatics* **73** (6) 334–339.

role as an adjunct to other antidepressant medication.[17] Good dietary sources of folic acid include dark green leafy vegetables, beans and pulses, and fortified breakfast cereals.

Serum zinc levels have been found to be significantly lower in majorly depressed subjects compared to normal controls and there is a negative correlation between zinc levels and severity of depression.[18] In a placebo-controlled zinc supplementation trial where zinc was given as an adjunct to standard antidepressant medication, it significantly reduced depression scores compared to the antidepressant plus placebo.[19] Good dietary sources of zinc include meat, shellfish, and bread and cereal products.

Nutrients and substance misuse behaviour

Where the relationship between nutrients and mood and behaviour in drug and alcohol users has been studied, the main focus has been on omega-3 PUFAs. It is thought that DHA might influence mood and behaviour through action on neurotransmitter systems since it is present in synaptic neuronal membranes, and EPA may affect neuronal function via neuroimmunological and vascular effects. It has been found that low levels of the neurotransmitters dopamine and serotonin, which are important for mood, are related to low levels of omega-3 fats in alcoholics, including those with a history of violent, impulsive behaviours.[20,21] An omega-3 double blind, placebo-controlled intervention study, involving drug users visiting a drug treatment clinic who were given a high daily dose of fish oil for three months, found a significant decrease in anger and anxiety in the fish oil group compared to controls.[22]

Relatively little research has looked at diet and drug-taking behaviour. A study using an animal model found that diets containing different types of

17   Taylor MJ, Carney S, Geddes J & Goodwin G (2003) Folate for depressive disorders. *Cochrane Database of Systematic Reviews* **2** CD003390.

18   Maes M, D'Haese PC, Scharpé S, D'Hondt P, Cosyns P & De Broe ME (1994) Hypozincemia in depression. *Journal of Affective Disorders* **31** (2) 135–140.

19   Novak G (2003) Effect of zinc supplementation on antidepressant therapy in unipolar depression: a preliminary placebo-controlled study. *Polish Journal of Pharmacology* **55** 1143–1147.

20   Hibbeln JR, Linnoila M, Umhau JC, Rawlings R, George DT & Salem N Jr (1998) Essential fatty acids predict metabolites of serotonin and dopamine in cerebrospinal fluid among healthy control subjects and early- and late-onset alcoholics. *Biological Psychiatry* **44** 235–242.

21   Hibbeln JR (1998) A replication study of violent and nonviolent subjects: cerebrospinal fluid metabolites of serotonin and dopamine are predicted by plasma essential fatty acids. *Biological Psychiatry* **44** 243–249.

22   Buydens-Branchey L, Branchey M & Hibbeln JR (2008) Associations between increases in plasma n-3 polyunsaturated fatty acids following supplementation and decreases in anger and anxiety in substance abusers. *Progress in Neuro-psychopharmacology and Biological Psychiatry* **32** (2) 568–575.

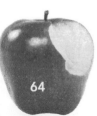

fatty acids could influence the levels of amphetamine-induced behaviour; trans-fatty acids were found to increase levels of hyperactivity as well as oxidative stress, when compared to omega-3 fatty acids.[23]

A small study of substance misusers in treatment found that those who did not relapse had significantly higher levels of DHA than those who did relapse.[24] In this study of 30, just under half dropped out, either just after entry into the study or after relapsing, leaving seven relapsers and 11 non-relapsers to complete the study.

Taking nutrient supplements

Virtually all intervention studies on mood and behaviour have been single nutrient interventions rather than whole diet interventions (the prison studies mentioned below being notable exceptions), since it is easier to set parameters and draw significant conclusions from such studies. However, it must again be stressed that whole balanced diets contain a full range of nutrients, some of which we might still not have discovered the importance of, and so the long-term aim must always be to achieve a balanced diet. When deciding whether to take nutrient supplements, the advice given earlier should be heeded, in that it is safer to take a multi-vitamin and mineral tablet at the level indicated on the packet, rather than take single vitamins and minerals, particularly at high levels.

Some of the more robust evidence for nutrients affecting mood comes from fish oil studies, and this may encourage drug and alcohol users to take fish oil supplements. Although fish oil studies have generally been carried out with negligible side effects – other than some upset stomachs resulting from the high levels of oil consumed – it should be noted that fish oil has anti-coagulant properties. Injecting drug users often suffer from thromboses and may be prescribed anticoagulant medication. Fish oil, and indeed many other nutrient supplements, can disrupt the effects of such medication. It should also be noted that these studies used high quality fish oil and *not* fish liver oil. It is important that fish liver oil (including cod liver oil) is not

23   Trevizol F, Benvegnú DM, Barcelos RC, Boufleur N, Dolci GS, Müller LG, Pase CS, Reckziegel P, Dias VT, Segat H, Teixeira AM, Emanuelli T, Rocha JB & Bürger ME (2010) Comparative study between n-6, trans and n-3 fatty acids on repeated amphetamine exposure: a possible factor for the development of mania. *Pharmacology,Biochemistry and Behavior* **97** (3) 560–565.

24   Buydens-Branchey L, Branchey M & Hibbeln JR (2009) Low plasma levels of docosahexaenoic acid are associated with an increased relapse vulnerability in substance abusers. *American Journal on Addictions* **18** 1–8.

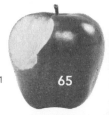

taken at quantities exceeding that stated on the packaging, since it contains vitamin A, which can be toxic at high levels. Advice should always be sought from a doctor if a person is being prescribed medication and is considering taking nutrient supplements.

Diet and drug users in prisons

Illicit drug use is still prevalent in prisons, although alcohol use may be less so, due to the difficulty in concealment. While some people will receive custodial sentences as a result of drug offences and continue drug use while in prison, others may initially take up drug use in prison as a means of dealing with their situation.

Drug-related health issues are commonplace in prisons. In men's prisons, an estimated nine per cent of the population has hepatitis C,[25] which is 20 times higher than the general population. The HIV rate for men in prison is estimated to be 15 times higher than the rate outside.[26] TB is also a concern. A study of individuals in London with TB showed the overall prevalence to be 27/100,000 with much higher rates among drug users (354/100,000) and prisoners (208/100,000),[27] possibly due to the confined conditions of communal drug-taking and the confined living space in prisons, although poor diet is also a factor in the progression of the disease. Oral health remains an issue for drug-using prisoners. In a study of French prisoners, which compared the oral health of heroin addict and non-addict prisoners, there were significantly higher levels of decayed, missing and filled teeth among the heroin addicts than non-addicts.[28] Mental health problems are common among prisoners and it is thought that there are currently more UK prisoners with mental health problems than ever before.[29]

Despite the physical and mental health concerns among prisoners, especially drug-using prisoners, relatively little emphasis has been placed

25 Prison Reform Trust & The National Aids Trust (2005) *HIV and Hepatitis in UK prisons: Addressing prisoners healthcare needs*. London: PRT and NAT.

26 Prison Reform Trust & The National Aids Trust (2005) *HIV and Hepatitis in UK prisons: Addressing prisoners healthcare needs*. London: PRT and NAT.

27 Story A, Murad S, Roberts W, Verheyen M & Hayward AC (2007) Tuberculosis in London: the importance of homelessness, problem drug use and prison. *Thorax* **62** 667–671.

28 Becart A (1997) The oral health status of drug addicts. A prison survey in Lille, France. *Journal of Forensic Odonto-Stomatology* **15** (2) 37–39.

29 The Bradley Report (2009) *Lord Bradley's review of people with mental health problems or learning disabilities in the criminal justice system*. London: Department of Health.

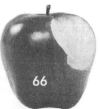

on improving diet in prisons. In 2008, the Associate Parliamentary Food and Health Forum recognised the mounting evidence supporting a link between diet and behaviour. This evidence included a rigorous double-blind placebo-controlled study in a young offenders' institute, which found that supplementation with vitamins, minerals and fatty acids resulted in 26.3% fewer offences in a treatment group than with a placebo control group.[30] A study in a Dutch prison showed a similar outcome.[31] With respect to prisons, the Health Forum recommended that:

'The National Offender Management Service (NOMS) gives serious consideration to any dietary intervention that can be used to improve the behaviour and mental well-being of offenders.

- *NOMS look positively at the case for introducing nutrient-based standards for meals in prisons, similar to those introduced for schools, but based on recommended daily intakes for adults.*

- *Effective measures should be taken in all prisons to inform prisoners about the benefits of a good diet and to persuade and encourage them to make healthy choices, both while they are in custody and after their release.'[32]*

The Food Standards Agency, under its former remit for healthy eating, introduced guidance for nutrient-based standards for meals served in institutions, including prisons. Within NOMS, the Integrated Drug Treatment System for Prisons (IDTS) has introduced basic healthy eating information for prisoners. The author has developed an evidence-based[33] healthy eating and well-being programme for the Ministry of Justice, to meet the needs of prisoners in drug treatment in English high security prisons, which has subsequently suffered at the hands of government cuts. Since then, two major reviews on mental health and drug treatment in the UK penal system – *The Bradley Report* and *The Patel Report* – made no mention of the diets of prisoners. Similarly, the British government's recent green paper on penal reform, *Breaking the Cycle: Effective punishment, rehabilitation and sentencing of offenders*, makes no mention at all of diet or healthy eating.

30   Gesch CB, Hammond SM, Hampson SE, Eves A & Crowder MJ (2002) Influence of supplementary vitamins, minerals and essential fatty acids on the antisocial behaviour of young adults. *British Journal of Psychiatry* **81** 22–28.

31   Zaalberg A, Nijman H, Bulten E, Stroosma L & van der Staak C (2009) Effects of nutritional supplements on aggression, rule-breaking, and psychopathology among young adult prisoners. *Aggressive Behavior* **35** 1–10.

32   Associate Parliamentary Food and Health Forum (2008) The Links between Diet and Behaviour: The links between diet and behaviour. London: FHF.

33   Sandwell HM & Wheatley M (2009) Healthy eating as part of drug treatment in prisons. *Prison Service Journal* **182** 15–26.

One of the current government's strategies for penal reform is to reduce the numbers of offenders with mental health and drug problems in the prison population, and instead treat them in the community, as recommended by the two mentioned reports. While this move is welcomed by many, there are some factors about a prison regime that could be viewed as a positive influence in attaining a balanced diet, and efforts should be encouraged to translate these into community treatment.

- Prisons have nutrient-based standards for food provision, which are unlikely to have been adopted by voluntary residential treatment centres that provide food for residents.

- Prisons provide three meals a day for prisoners, often providing the most balanced diets drug users will have received for some time. Such consistent and reasonably balanced diets may not be achieved by individuals living alone in the community while attending community-based treatment programmes.

- The pre-selection of meals from menus in prisons allows prisoners to make healthy choices in advance, rather than making impulse purchases of food when hungry.

- Prisoners may have the opportunity to learn about healthy eating and learn cooking skills, through education and training, which may not be offered to them in the community.

- Prisoners in drug treatment programmes are encouraged to take up physical activity and have access to free PE facilities, as this is known to support recovery from drug use. This is less likely to occur in community treatment programmes.

How improving diet could help in recovery

A role for drug treatment providers

Despite the lack of research studies specifically looking at how diet affects mood and behaviour in drug users, it is possible to make some logical assumptions based on what is known about the link between diet, mood and behaviour; mood, behaviour and drug use; mood and physical health; physical health and drug use (see Figure 3.4).

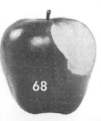

Figure 3.4: How diet could help improve the physical and mental health of drug and alcohol users

Malnutrition can negatively impact on mood and behaviour

Improving diet can help improve physical health

Those who misuse drugs and alcohol are often malnourished

Poor physical health can negatively impact on mood

Improving the diet of drug and alcohol users could benefit their physical and mental health

Low levels of specific nutrients are associated with negative mood and behaviour

Those who misuse drugs and alcohol and develop dependencies often have poor physical health related to their dependency

Those who misuse drugs and alcohol and develop dependencies are likely to have an underlying mood disorder and mental health problems

Specific nutrients can positively modify mood and behaviour

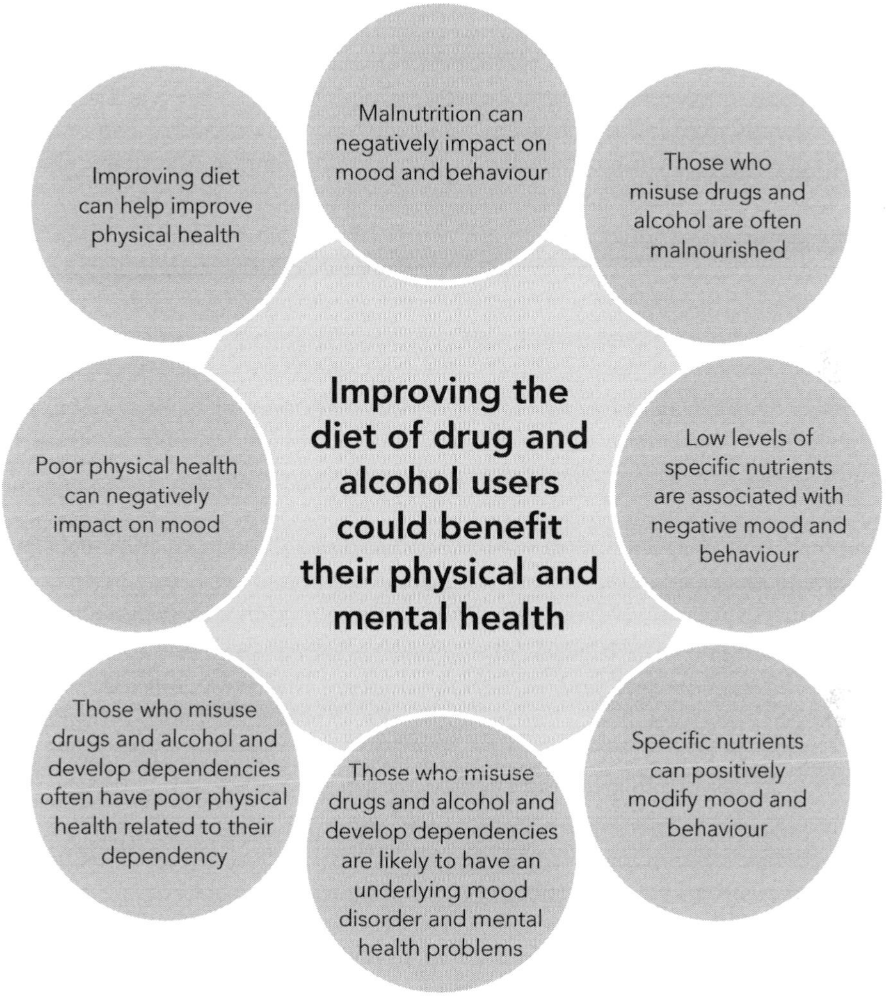

It is important for drug and alcohol treatment providers to include healthy eating as an integral part of their treatment programme. They can help improve their clients' diets by providing:

■ healthy, balanced meals based on the Eatwell Plate model

■ information, advice and encouragement in making healthy food choices

■ the teaching of cooking, shopping and even growing skills, or by being able to refer clients to suitable education programmes

■ encouragement to develop the social aspects and pleasure of food eg. planning, shopping, cooking and eating a meal together.

Other lifestyle considerations

When an individual has reached the point in their life when they are ready to give up drugs, they may well also be in a state of mind to improve other elements of their life such as food choices and activity levels. Wherever possible, improvements in diet should always be considered in the context of improving the person's entire lifestyle. Physical activity is an important factor and one that is often overlooked by drug treatment providers. Physical activity can help with depression, anxiety, increasing energy, building self-worth, and improving sleep quality[34]. Physical exercise does not have to be expensive. Outdoor activities such as running, walking and cycling, are free (once the basic equipment has been acquired) and all are suitable as group activities that could be integrated into treatment programmes.

Sleep quality is another important factor contributing to mood, since poor or inadequate sleep can cause irritability and stress. People who have problems with sleep are at an increased risk of developing emotional disorders, depression, and anxiety. Dietary factors may influence sleep quality, for example, a heavy, protein and fat-rich meal late at night may disrupt sleep, since a relatively long time is required to digest and absorb protein and fat. The old adage that eating cheese before bed gives you nightmares may hold some truth in that mature cheeses are rich in tyramine, which can disrupt sleep, raise blood pressure and induce sweating, palpitations and migraines in some people. Caffeine can also disrupt sleep by blocking the action of adenosine, a substance in the body which inhibits neuronal activity and induces sleep. In some people this effect is much greater than in others since people metabolise caffeine at different rates, and the time of day to cease caffeine consumption to benefit sleep can vary from person to person. It is commonly reported that individuals in treatment and recovery often drink copious cups of strong (and highly sugared) coffee. Such levels of caffeine could be contributing to sleep disruption, increased levels of anxiety or irritability, and low mood, none of which are helpful for those aiming to remain on an even keel and be drug-free.

---

34   Fox KR (1999) The influence of physical activity on mental well-being. *Public Health Nutrition* **2** (3a) 411–418.

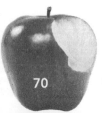

Finally, daily exposure to sunlight is another important lifestyle factor often neglected by those working in the drug treatment field and medical profession. In northern Europe, the absence of daylight of sufficient wavelength during the shorter days of the winter months is a major factor behind seasonal affective disorder (SAD), highlighting the importance of daylight during the remainder of the year – late spring, summer and early autumn months. Vitamin D, produced by the skin in response to sunlight during these months, is now thought to play a role in mental health. As well as being important for bone health, muscle strength and immunity, vitamin D deficiency has been linked to an increased incidence of depression and schizophrenia.[35] In the UK, no vitamin D is made by the skin between October and March, and during the remainder of the year it is recommended that we have 20 minutes of unprotected sunlight a day (more for darker skins) to ensure that sufficient vitamin D is made by the skin (avoiding times when the sun is at its strongest and may burn). The major dietary sources of vitamin D are oily fish and liver, and there is also some in milk, eggs and some fortified products such as breakfast cereals and vegetable oil spreads.

Both vitamin D supplements[36] and UV light therapy[37] have been shown to have a positive effect on mood. Low vitamin D levels are a problem for the UK population in general, especially since the main dietary sources tend not be popular and because of a tendency to overprotect the skin in summer. These problems are likely to be exacerbated in drug and alcohol users who are often malnourished and may lead a largely indoor lifestyle. During treatment and recovery, it is important to encourage individuals to spend time outdoors, preferably engaged in a physical leisure activity.

Having a balanced diet, doing exercise, exposing the skin to sunshine and maintaining quality sleep are simple lifestyle changes that could be encouraged and would enhance any treatment programme. In doing so, treatment providers could help imprint new, more positive lifestyle patterns on individuals undergoing treatment.

35   Hollick MF (2007) Vitamin D deficiency. *New England Journal of Medicine* **357** (3) 266–281.

36   Lansdowne ATG & Provost SC (1998) Vitamin D3 enhances mood in healthy subjects during winter. *Psychopharmacology (Berlin)* **135** (3) 19–323.

37   Feldman SR, Liguori A, Kucenic M, Rapp SR, Fleischer AB Jr, Lang W & Kaur M (2004) Ultraviolet exposure is a reinforcing stimulus in frequent indoor tanners. *Journal of the American Academy of Dermatology* **51** 45–51.

Further reading and resources

Associate Parliamentary Food and Health Forum (2008) *The Links between Diet and Behaviour.* London: FHR. Available at: http://www.fhf.org.uk/meetings/inquiry2007/FHF_inquiry_report_diet_and_behaviour.pdf (accessed July 2011).

Department of Health (2010) *The Patel Report: Reducing drug-related crime and rehabilitating offenders.* London: Department of Health Prison Drug Treatment Strategy Review Group.

Lord Bradley (2009) *The Bradley Report: Lord Bradley's review of people with mental health problems or learning disabilities in the criminal justice system.* London: Department of Health.

Ministry of Justice (2010) *Breaking the Cycle: Effective punishment, rehabilitation and sentencing of offenders.* Available at: http://www.justice. gov.uk/consultations/docs/breaking-the-cycle.pdf (accessed September 2011).

Prison Service Journal (March 2009) *Special edition focusing on diet in UK prisons. Issue 182.* Published by HM Prison Service.

Useful websites

British Liver Trust has information and publications about liver disease. www.britishlivertrust.org.uk

Council for the Homeless Northern Ireland (CHNI) produces various resources for those working with the homeless, including Nutrition for Alcohol Users. www.chni.org.uk.

Food Matters provides food and well-being training for organisations dealing with vulnerable adults. www.foodmatters.org

The Hepatitis C Trust has information including eating advice for individuals living with hepatitis C. www.hepctrust.org.uk.

Prison Reform Trust produces various publications concerning topics around penal reform. www.prisonreformtrust.org.uk.

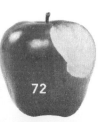

Chapter 4

Food addiction: fact or fiction?

Jane Nodder

Introduction

Food addiction is a controversial topic that regularly receives media attention. Patients often say they are 'addicted' to certain foods, with chocolate, bread, sugar, wheat and dairy products being the common culprits. They may 'use' such foods to cope with stress, anxiety or feelings of inadequacy, or because of the palatability of foods that are rich in sugar, salt or fat, or against a background of food restriction or environmental conditioning. Some people develop chaotic eating patterns or eating disorders characterised by feeling out of control around food, being trapped in a cycle of compulsive or binge eating, and are unable to adhere to a nutritional programme. These characteristics can contribute to the patient's sense of 'food addiction'. Over time, such behaviour can also be detrimental to health as persistently eating and eating larger meals or the 'wrong' foods can lead to weight gain, obesity, malnutrition and related problems.

But does food really create an addiction process in a similar way to other addictive substances? This chapter attempts to marry research findings regarding food addiction with the patient perspective and considers how simple nutritional interventions might be included in approaches to managing food addiction and disordered eating patterns.

The nature of food addiction

- The concept of food addiction is controversial due to difficulties with definitions and a lack of rigorous scientific data.
- Excessive eating has been associated with addictive personality characteristics and can co-exist with drug and alcohol addiction; however, it is unlikely that all instances of excess food consumption can be considered as addictive behaviour.

Unlike other potentially addictive substances, food is essential for survival. We need to eat repeatedly every day and it is 'normal' to look forward to eating to provide energy, gain essential nutrients and receive pleasure. The term 'food addiction' indicates a biochemical state that creates a physiological craving for certain foods that has been described as being comparable to the cravings some people experience for alcohol and other substances.[1] However, food addiction is not yet included in the *Diagnostic and Statistical Manual of Mental Disorders* (DSM-IV-TR),[2] and as a concept it has been historically controversial due to difficulties with definitions and a lack of rigorous scientific data.

Excessive eating is characteristic of eating disorders such as bulimia nervosa and binge eating disorder, which have also been associated with addictive personality characteristics. Indeed, many binge eaters would meet some, if not all, of the DSM-IV-TR (2000) criteria for substance dependence at the peak of their illness.[3] Dysfunctional eating patterns and excessive weight gain can also be co-morbid with drug and alcohol addiction. Men have described how binge eating and food seem to substitute drug use and satisfy cravings in early recovery, only to be replaced by concerns for weight gain in mid to late recovery.[4] Although it may not be appropriate to include all instances of excess food consumption under addictive behaviour, considering each addictive condition separately may hinder a more comprehensive view.[5,6]

Possible mechanisms of food addiction

- Neurotransmitters and the brain's reward system are implicated in both food and other addictions mainly through the dopamine, opiate and glutamate systems.

- Some individuals may actually need more food to obtain a sense of pleasure and reward; reward deficiency syndrome is characterised by a reduced number and sensitivity of dopamine receptors.

1   Sheppard K (2000) *From the First Bite: A complete guide to recovery from food addiction*. US: Health Communications.

2   American Psychiatric Association (2000) *Diagnostic and Statistical Manual. 4th edition text revision (TR)*. Washington DC: American Psychiatric Association.

3   Cassin SE & von Ranson KM (2007) Is binge eating experienced as an addiction? *Appetite* **49** (3) 687–690.

4   Cowan J & Devine C (2008) Food, eating, and weight concerns of men in recovery from substance addiction. *Appetite* **50** (1) 33–42.

5   Adam TC & Epel ES (2007) Stress, eating and the reward system. *Physiology & Behaviour* **91**(4) 449–458.

6   Pelchat ML (2009) Food addiction in humans. *Journal of Nutrition* **139** 620–602.

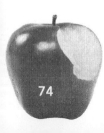

- Some potential addictive properties have been shown for foods rich in sugar, fat and salt, which may promote 'addiction-like' behaviour and neuronal change under certain conditions.

- Other factors that may play a role in food addiction include gender, learned expectation and alternating dietary access and restriction.

Despite the evidence for the involvement of a range of factors, many researchers believe that true addiction requires a psychoactive substance, which produces symptoms such as physical tolerance and withdrawal. Recently, there have been further attempts to examine the connections between food and chemical, physiological and psychological dependence, and to determine whether the concept of food addiction is meaningful and, if it is, how it should be addressed and by whom.

Reward and pleasure pathways

Food intake is regulated by two complementary drives: the *homeostatic pathway* that controls energy balance by increasing our motivation to eat following depletion of energy stores, and the *hedonic (reward-based) pathway*, which increases our desire for highly palatable foods and can override the homeostatic pathway where energy is abundant. In contrast, the motivation to use drugs is mediated only by the reward pathway.

Repeated stimulation of reward pathways may lead to neurobiological adaptations that promote the compulsive nature of overeating. Neurotransmitters and the brain's reward system are implicated in both food and other addictions, mainly through the release of dopamine in both the nucleus accumbens and the dorsal striatum areas of the brain.[7,8] Sugar has been shown to promote addiction-like behaviour and neuronal change under certain conditions. For example, rats given an opioid antagonist demonstrated behavioural and neurochemical signs of opioid withdrawal with a repeated, excessive intake of sugar,[9] while rats given intermittent access to sucrose following deprivation, progressively increased their intake and dopamine release, compared to three control groups.[10] Motivation for sugar

7   Adam TC & Epel ES (2007) Stress, eating and the reward system. *Physiology & Behaviour* **91** (4) 449–458.

8   Volkow ND, Wang GJ, Fowler JS, Thanos PP, Logan J, Gatley SJ, Gifford A, Ding YS, Wong C & Pappas N (2002) Brain DA D2 receptors predict reinforcing effects of stimulants in humans: replication study. *Synapse* **46** (2) 79–82.

9   Colantuoni C, Rada P, McCarthy J, Patten C, Avena NM, Chadeayne A & Hoebel BG (2002) Evidence that intermittent, excessive sugar intake causes endogenous opioid dependence. *Obesity Research* **10** (6) 478–488.

10   Rada P, Avena NM & Hoebel BG (2005) Daily bingeing on sugar repeatedly releases dopamine in the accumbens shell. *Neuroscience* **134** (3) 737–744.

also increased when it was removed from animals with sufficient experience of it.[11] In food-deprived human subjects, the dopamine reward system can be triggered merely by the sight or smell of food, whether or not the food is eaten, [12] and elevated cortisol may also influence the reward value of food.[13]

Some individuals may actually need more food to obtain a sense of pleasure and reward. Reward deficiency syndrome, characterised by a reduced number and sensitivity of dopamine receptors, has been identified in obesity, binge eating disorder and bulimia nervosa, and may be linked to changes in individual gene markers.[14] Furthermore, those parts of the brain responsible for pleasure sensation in the mouth, lips and tongue have been found to be more active in the obese, compared with normal weight controls, and may increase an individual's sensitivity to the rewarding properties of food.[15]

Opioid release, regulatory feedback and glutamate receptors

Palatable foods have been shown to stimulate the opiate system in the brain via the hypothalamic pituitary axis[16,17] and the digestion of food proteins such as casein and gluten may also stimulate the production of opioid peptides. These substances can exert an addictive, drug-like effect, and it has been suggested that individuals may consume foods containing these proteins to maintain the production of opioid peptides and avoid symptoms of withdrawal.[18]

Deficiencies in regulatory feedback substances produced in the bowel have also been associated with cravings and compulsive eating.[19] Glutamate receptors, involved in other types of addiction, may also play a role (see Chapter 2).[20]

11   Avena NM, Rada P & Hoebel BG (2009) Sugar and fat bingeing have notable differences in addictive-like behaviour. *Journal of Nutrition* **139** 623–628.

12   Volkow ND, Wang GJ, Fowler JS, Thanos PP, Logan J, Gatley SJ, Gifford A, Ding YS, Wong C & Pappas N (2002) Brain DA D2 receptors predict reinforcing effects of stimulants in humans: replication study. *Synapse* **46** (2) 79–82.

13   Adam TC & Epel ES (2007) Stress, eating and the reward system. *Physiology & Behaviour* **91** (4) 449–458.

14   Davis C, Levitan RD, Kaplan AS, Carter J, Reid C, Curtis C, Patte K, Hwang R & Kennedy JL (2008) Reward sensitivity and the D2 dopamine receptor gene: A case-control study of binge eating disorder. *Progress in Neuropsychopharmacology and Biological Psychiatry* **32** (3) 620–628.

15   Wang GJ, Volkow ND, Felder C, Fowler JS, Levy AV, Pappas NR, Wong CT, Zhu W & Netusil N (2002) Enhanced resting activity of the oral somatosensory cortex in obese subjects. *Neuroreport* **13** (9) 1151–1155.

16   Adam TC & Epel ES (2007) Stress, eating and the reward system. *Physiology & Behaviour* **91** (4) 449–458.

17   Pelchat ML (2009) Food addiction in humans. *Journal of Nutrition* **139** 620–622.

18   Mercer ME & Holder MD (1997) Food cravings, endogenous opioid peptides, and food intake: a review. *Appetite* **29** (3) 325–352

19   Pelchat ML (2009) Food addiction in humans. *Journal of Nutrition* **139** 620–622.

20   Kalivas PW (2009) The glutamate homeostasis hypothesis of addiction. *Nature Reviews Neuroscience* **10** (8) 561–572.

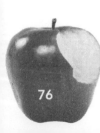

Gender

Women may find it more difficult than men to control food intake, possibly due to the influence of female sex hormones. 'Addiction' to carbohydrate foods has also attracted particular interest with regard to women. Self-identified female carbohydrate cravers appeared to over-consume carbohydrates, leading to weight gain,[21] and female carbohydrate cravers also chose a carbohydrate beverage significantly more often than a protein-rich beverage when rendered mildly distressed.[22] In addition, the carbohydrate beverage was perceived as more palatable and produced greater mood improvement in carbohydrate cravers than in independent pre-trial taste testers. 90% of female college students, compared with 53% of males, also indicated increased cravings for carbohydrate foods high in fat with negative mood.[23]

Other factors

Some researchers believe that results from animal models can be extrapolated to humans and are crucial to understanding the mechanisms and biological process of food addiction.[24] Others consider that there is no support from human literature for a physical addiction to foods such as sugar, or a role for sugar addiction in eating disorders,[25] and no explanation for theories that chocolate, for example, has a particular appeal to women.[26] Their view is that learned expectations are important alongside any biological effect of a particular food (eg. eating sugar is naturally pleasurable and teaches an individual to desire it) and that such expectations can therefore be unlearned. Food is also not generally seen as comparable to other addictions as it does not fit the 'use', 'abstinence', 'relapse' model of substance use.[27] Addictive eating patterns may arise more from food being consumed against a background of alternating dietary access and restriction that places the body in caloric deficit and contributes to poor nutritional status, than from the sensory properties of food itself.[28]

21   Spring B, Schneider K, Smith M, Kendzor D, Appelhans B, Hedeker D & Pagoto S (2008) Abuse potential of carbohydrates for overweight carbohydrate cravers. *Psychopharmacology (Berl)* **197** (4) 637–647.

22   Corsica JA & Spring BJ (2008) Carbohydrate craving: a double-blind, placebo-controlled test of the self-medication hypothesis. *Eating Behaviors* **9** (4) 447–454.

23   Christensen L & Pettijohn L (2001) Mood and carbohydrate cravings. *Appetite* **36** (2) 137–145.

24   Corwin RL & Grigson PS. (2009) Symposium overview: food addiction: fact or fiction? *Journal of Nutrition* **139** (3) 617–619.

25   Benton D (2009) The plausibility of sugar addiction and its role in obesity and eating disorders. *Clinical Nutrition* **29** (3) 288–303.

26   Rabinerson D & Melamed N (2009) 'On bitter and sweet': women and chocolate. *Harefuah* **48** (8) 539–542, 570–571.

27   Corwin RL & Grigson PS (2009) Symposium overview: food addiction: fact or fiction? *Clinical Nutrition* **139** (3) 617–619.

28   Pelchat ML (2009) Food addiction in humans. *Journal of Nutrition* **139** 620–622.

Food addiction and DSM-IV-TR (2000): criteria for substance dependence

■ Food can be considered as a potentially addictive substance for review against the seven DSM-IV-TR (2000) criteria (tolerance, withdrawal, loss of control, reducing intake, time consumption, effect on other activities and persistent use) for diagnosing substance dependence eg. for alcohol and drugs.

Table 4.1 shows the seven criteria the DSM-IV-TR (2000) sets out for diagnosing substance dependence eg. for alcohol and drugs, with an individual needing to meet at least three criteria in the same year for a diagnosis.[29] Another approach for reviewing the concept of food as an addictive substance is therefore to consider food as a potentially addictive substance against these same seven criteria.[30]

Tolerance

Rats have been shown to increase their intake of sugar during a trial period and to exhibit neurochemical changes indicative of sensitisation or tolerance.[31,32,33] In humans, 49.4% of binge-eating participants identified tolerance and the need to consume increasing amounts of binge food to gain the desired effect on mood,[34] while individuals with bulimia nervosa ate more food, more often and for longer periods, and felt increasingly out of control as their illness progressed.[35] Again, carbohydrate foods are often positioned as the main possible culprits regarding tolerance, and abstinence from sugar and high fat foods is frequently recommended in popular websites and self-help literature relating to food addiction.

29   American Psychiatric Association (2000) *Diagnostic and Statistical Manual. 4th Edition Text Revision (TR)*. Washington DC: American Psychiatric Association.

30   Sheppard K (2000) *From the First Bite: A complete guide to recovery from food addiction*. US: Health Communications.

31   Colantuoni C, Rada P, McCarthy J, Patten C, Avena NM, Chadeayne A & Hoebel BG (2002) Evidence that intermittent, excessive sugar intake causes endogenous opioid dependence. *Obesity Research* **10** (6) 478–488.

32   Avena NM, Rada P & Hoebel BG (2009) Sugar and fat bingeing have notable differences in addictive-like behaviour. *Journal of Nutrition* **139** 623–628.

33   Rada P, Avena NM & Hoebel BG (2005) Daily bingeing on sugar repeatedly releases dopamine in the accumbens shell. *Neuroscience* **134** (3) 737–744.

34   Cassin SE & von Ranson KM (2007) Is binge eating experienced as an addiction? *Appetite* **49** (3) 687–690.

35   Colles SL, Dixon JB & O'Brien PE (2008) Loss of control is central to psychological disturbance associated with binge eating disorder. *Obesity* **16** (3) 608–614.

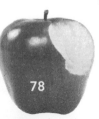

Table 4.1: Criteria for substance dependence	
1. Tolerance	Need for considerably increased amounts of a substance to achieve intoxication or a desired effect, or a notably reduced effect from continued use of the same amount of a substance
2. Withdrawal	Characteristic withdrawal symptoms for a substance, or use of the same, or a very similar substance, to relieve or avoid withdrawal symptoms
3. Loss of control	Substance is often taken in larger amounts or over a longer period than intended
4. Reducing intake	Individual experiences a persistent desire, or unsuccessful efforts, to eliminate or reduce substance use
5. Time consumption	Great deal of time is spent obtaining and using the substance, or recovering from its effects
6. Effect on other activities	Other important activities (social, occupational, or recreational) are affected as a result of substance use
7. Persistent use	Individual continues to use a substance despite knowing that such use is likely to cause, or exacerbate, physical or psychological problems
Adapted from American Psychiatric Association (2000) *Diagnostic and Statistical Manual (4th Text Revision)* (TR). Washington DC: APA.	

Withdrawal

Sugar-dependent rats experienced signs and symptoms synonymous with drug withdrawal when sugar was removed from their diets and had imbalances in brain chemistry that were qualitatively similar to withdrawal from morphine and nicotine.[36,37,38] In humans, cravings after abstinence also seem to be symptomatic of sugar withdrawal, while withdrawal from a high sugar diet and a high fat diet resulted in neurochemical responses and a depressed state that appeared comparable to drug withdrawal.

---

36   Colantuoni C, Rada P, McCarthy J, Patten C, Avena NM, Chadeayne A & Hoebel BG (2002) Evidence that intermittent , excessive sugar intake causes endogenous opioid dependence. *Obesity Research* **10** (6) 478–488.

37   Avena NM, Rada P, Hoebel BG (2009) Sugar and fat bingeing have notable differences in addictive-like behaviour. *Journal of Nutrition* **139** 623–8.

38   Rada P, Avena NM & Hoebel BG (2005) Daily bingeing on sugar repeatedly releases dopamine in the accumbens shell. *Neuroscience* **134** (3) 737–744.

67.1% of binge eating participants identified withdrawal symptoms such as restlessness, irritability, headaches and insomnia if they were unable to binge,[39] while self-reported carbohydrate cravers felt anxious, fatigued and depressed prior to cravings, compared to satisfied and happy following carbohydrate consumption.[40] 'Chocoholics' refrained from reducing their chocolate intake due to the fear of experiencing withdrawal symptoms and described their sense of *'feeling out of control, angry and depressed'* and their need to *'give in to their cravings'* if denied chocolate.[41]

Loss of control

92.4% of participants with binge eating disorder stated that they tried to stay in control of their food intake to reduce their binge eating,[42] and loss of control also seemed closely related to psychological markers of distress eg. depression, and increased binge frequency and size.[43] Elevated cortisol levels have also been identified in binge eaters, indicating a degree of stress which may impact an individual's ability to control their food intake.[44]

Reducing intake

Compared to obese and normal weight controls, individuals with binge eating disorder frequently describe a persistent desire, or unsuccessful efforts, to cut their use of food, but experience difficulty actually reducing their intake. 83.5% of participants with binge eating disorder (BED) felt unable to control or reduce binges,[45] and self-identified food addicts also described a wide range of failed attempts to eat less.[46]

Time requirements

Obtaining and using food takes on extreme importance in both binge eating disorder and bulimia nervosa, with individuals also spending a lot

39   Cassin SE & von Ranson KM (2007) Is binge eating experienced as an addiction? *Appetite* **49** (3) 687–690.

40   Christensen L & Pettijohn L (2001) Mood and carbohydrate cravings. *Appetite* **36** (2) 137–145.

41   Benford R & Gough B (2006) Defining and defending 'unhealthy' practices: a discourse analysis of chocolate 'addicts' accounts. *Journal of Health Psychology* **11** (3) 427–440.

42   Cassin SE & von Ranson KM (2007) Is binge eating experienced as an addiction? *Appetite* **49** (3) 687–690.

43   Colles SL, Dixon JB & O'Brien PE (2008) Loss of control is central to psychological disturbance associated with binge eating disorder. *Obesity* **16** (3) 608–614.

44   Gluck ME (2006) Stress response and binge eating disorder. *Appetite* **46** (1) 26–30.

45   Cassin SE & von Ranson KM (2007) Is binge eating experienced as an addiction? *Appetite* **49** (3) 687–690.

46   Ifland JR, Preuss HG, Marcus MT, Rourke KM, Taylor WC, Burau K, Jacobs WS, Kadish W & Manso G (2009) Refined food addiction: a classic substance use disorder. *Medical Hypotheses* **72** (5) 518–526.

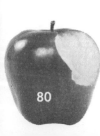

of time dealing with the emotional consequences of excess, often secretive and shameful, food consumption.[47] 59.5% of participants with binge eating disorder identified with the issues relating to time taken to obtain and use food,[48] and self-identified food addicts described being in and out of the kitchen all day, getting up at night to eat and spending a lot of time buying and eating food and 'sleeping off' binges.[49]

Effect on other activities

Linked to time requirements, 48.1% of BED participants described how the drive to consume refined high sugar foods was stronger than the drive to choose other important social, occupational, or recreational activities.[50] Obese individuals have been described as working significantly harder to obtain refined snacks compared with lean participants, even when the alternative is pleasurable sedentary activity.[51]

Persistent use

A very high percentage (91.1%) of participants with binge eating disorder continued to use food even when they recognised that they were experiencing ongoing physical or psychological problems that may well have been caused or exacerbated by their use of food.[52] Furthermore, associating a diet high in calories and refined food with obesity, heart disease and diabetes did not appear to deter self-reported, refined food addicts from binge eating.[53] Binge eating may provide sufficient temporary, short-term relief from psychological distress for individuals to disregard the potential risks to health and tolerate the rapid deterioration in mood, guilt and self-disgust that follows a period of excessive eating. Reward deficiency syndrome may also contribute to the persistent use of food.[54]

47   Colles SL, Dixon JB & O'Brien PE (2008) Loss of control is central to psychological disturbance associated with binge eating disorder. *Obesity* **16** (3) 608–614.

48   Cassin SE & von Ranson KM (2007) Is binge eating experienced as an addiction? *Appetite* **49** (3) 687–690.

49   Ifland JR, Preuss HG, Marcus MT, Rourke KM, Taylor WC, Burau K, Jacobs WS, Kadish W & Manso G (2009) Refined food addiction: a classic substance use disorder. *Medical Hypotheses* **72** (5) 518–526.

50   Cassin SE & von Ranson KM (2007) Is binge eating experienced as an addiction? *Appetite* **49** (3) 687–690.

51   Epstein LH, Temple JL, Neaderhiser BJ, Salis RJ, Erbe RW & Leddy JJ (2007) Food reinforcement, the dopamine D2 receptor genotype, and energy intake in obese and nonobese humans. *Behavioral Neuroscience* **121** (5) 877–886.

52   Cassin SE & von Ranson KM (2007) Is binge eating experienced as an addiction? *Appetite* 8 (3) 687–690.

53   Ifland JR, Preuss HG, Marcus MT, Rourke KM, Taylor WC, Burau K, Jacobs WS, Kadish W & Manso G (2009) Refined food addiction: a classic substance use disorder. *Medical Hypotheses* **72** (5) 518–526.

54   Davis C, Levitan RD, Kaplan AS, Carter J, Reid C, Curtis C, Patte K, Hwang R & Kennedy JL (2008) Reward sensitivity and the D2 dopamine receptor gene: A case-control study of binge eating disorder. *Progress in Neuropsychopharmacology and Biological Psychiatry* **32** (3) 620–628.

Using evidence to inform clinical practice

- The neurobiological evidence for food addiction is compelling.

- There is also some, although probably not sufficient, evidence for food addiction when comparing food as a potential substance for dependence against the seven DSM-IV-TR (2000) criteria.

- Nevertheless, clinicians can still use the current research evidence to offer individualised practical help and support to people who report food addiction.

To summarise, from a research perspective, the neurobiological evidence for food addiction is compelling with accumulating evidence to suggest a similar impact on the brain from both food and classic drugs, but with weaker effects for food. Against the DSM-IV-TR (2000) criteria there is also substantial evidence that some individuals lose control over food consumption, repeatedly fail to reduce intake and have difficulty abstaining from, or reducing, consumption of certain foods even with knowledge of possible negative consequences. However, there is probably not sufficient evidence to classify food as an addictive substance according to all seven DSM-IV-TR (2000) criteria. In particular, more research is needed with regard to the criteria relating to tolerance and withdrawal; the time spent obtaining, using and recovering from excess food consumption; and the degree to which important activities are given up due to overconsumption of food.

Nevertheless, individual patients still describe an 'addiction' to certain foods and report a strong need to eat more of these foods to 'get a lift' and withdrawal symptoms when cutting down consumption. Addictive overeating seems therefore to be not just a 'theoretical construct', but something that truly resonates with people's actual experience, and a potential disorder that clinicians need to accept and be confident to work with.[55]

So how might clinicians use the current research evidence to offer practical help and support to people who report food addiction? When working with such patients it would seem important to:

- recognise that addictive overeating is a very real experience for certain people and manage each patient as an individual

---

55 Schroder R, Sellman D & Elmslie J (2010) Addictive overeating: lessons learned from medical students' perceptions of Overeaters Anonymous. *Journal of the New Zealand Medical Association* **123** (1311) 15–21.

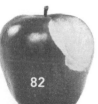

■ understand that in binge eating disorder, bulimia nervosa and obesity patients experience a loss of control characteristic of substance addiction

■ remember that food intake is regulated by both the homeostatic and the reward pathways, and that in binge eating the consumption of highly-refined foods involves the dopamine reward pathway, and possibly also the opiate and glutamate pathways

■ consider that highly palatable foods may not be addictive per se, but can become so following a restriction/binge pattern of consumption

■ explore the use of questionnaires such as the Yale Food Addiction Scale (currently in development) to help patients with possible food addiction and eating difficulties with losing weight, and offer support and advice for weight loss and weight loss maintenance issues linked to 'food addiction'

■ educate patients regarding the potential role of refined sugars and fats in food addiction

■ modify the stress response in eating pathologies through diet.

Nutritional approaches

■ A range of simple nutritional interventions involving macro and micronutrients can be considered to restore individual, biochemical imbalance and support recovery from food 'addiction'.

In addition to the strategies outlined above, a qualified nutrition professional can introduce simple nutritional approaches using the checklists shown in Tables 4.1 and 4.2 (see Appendix to this chapter), to manage symptoms associated with withdrawal, and support key biochemical imbalances during recovery from food addiction. Such approaches include the following.

■ Using a food plan to structure eating patterns to encourage either three meals with two/three snacks, or four/five small meals, at three-to-four-hour intervals throughout the day, starting with the individual's current eating pattern and making gradual but steady changes.

■ Balancing food intake for complex carbohydrates, protein and fats by aiming for 45–55% of calories from carbohydrate, 20–25% from protein and 25–30% from fat[56] based on 1,500–2,500 calories as appropriate for the individual; any nutritional approach must protect against under and overeating and recognise that it can be difficult to meet basic nutrient needs below 1,500 calories per day.[57]

---

56 Herrin M (2003) *Nutrition Counselling in the Treatment of Eating Disorders*. NY: Brunner Routledge.
57 Herrin M (2003) *Nutrition Counselling in the Treatment of Eating Disorders*. NY: Brunner Routledge.

- Depending on size and weight, including 20–30g of protein containing all essential amino acids at each meal to help reduce any cravings for refined carbohydrates [60]; for example: three medium eggs, a small can (100g) of tuna, 150g cottage cheese, small matchbox-sized piece (40g) of cheddar cheese, 600ml semi-skimmed or skimmed milk, 6–8 tablespoons of beans, lentils or chickpeas, two medium slices (75g) meat, one small (75g) breast of chicken, one medium (100g) fillet of fish, 250g of tofu.

- Ensuring a daily intake of essential omega fatty acids from oily fish, nuts and seeds to support neurotransmitter function and help with symptoms of low mood, depression and hormone imbalance.

- Eating a wide range of vegetables, and two to three servings of fruit per day for carbohydrate, fibre, essential vitamins, minerals and phytonutrients for metabolic function.

- Adding foods containing the amino acid tryptophan (eg. milk, poultry, eggs, red meats, soybeans, tofu and almonds) to try to support serotonin production and mood.

- Obtaining up to 1,500mg/day of calcium from foods such as dairy products, green leafy vegetables, soya products, canned fish and supplements.[58]

- Ensuring adequate total fluid intake of 1.2–1.5 litres fluid/day.

- Reducing sugars, refined foods and stimulants to support blood glucose control, insulin management and mood, but without focusing on 'forbidden' foods;[59,60] for food 'addicts' avoiding certain foods can only increase their desirability and raise fears that the individual will eventually succumb to the very foods they are trying to avoid; including some 'fun food' as part of a daily food plan can help to legitimise all foods.[61]

Nutrition counselling can be included alongside other therapeutic work in either a group or an individual setting. Sessions could initially run weekly, moving to fortnightly or monthly according to need. Individuals should leave each nutritional counselling session with a realistic goal to work on, and be encouraged to keep full records of food intake linked to mood/ emotions/situations between sessions for review at subsequent visits.

58   Herrin M (2003) *Nutrition Counselling in the Treatment of Eating Disorders*. NY: Brunner Routledge.

59   Herrin M (2003) *Nutrition Counselling in the Treatment of Eating Disorders*. NY: Brunner Routledge.

60   American Dietetic Association & Position of the American Dietetic Association (2006) Nutrition intervention in the treatment of anorexia nervosa, bulimia nervosa, and other eating disorders. *Journal of the American Dietetic Association* **106** (12) 2073–2082.

61   Herrin M (2003) *Nutrition Counselling in the Treatment of Eating Disorders*. NY: Brunner Routledge.

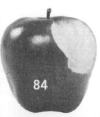

Conclusion

By accepting that food addiction is a very real experience for some people, clinicians can use current research evidence to offer practical strategies and simple nutritional interventions to restore individual, biochemical imbalance and support recovery.

With acknowledgement to Madeleine Weaver, BSc Health Sciences, Nutritional Therapy, for her undergraduate work on food addiction.

Appendix

Nutritional approaches checklists

Tables 4.1 and 4.2 provide checklists of possible nutritional approaches for addressing food addiction. These checklists can be used by a nutrition professional or an individual patient as a guide for planning actions relating to dietary changes over a period of time. For example, appropriate dietary goals for a first consultation with a nutrition professional, or the first week of an individual identifying dietary changes for themselves, might include addressing intake of complex carbohydrates, protein and vitamin D. The checklist would prompt a nutrition professional, or an individual, to think about their current carbohydrate intake in terms of the balance between complex and simple, high and low glycaemic index (GI) and sources of carbohydrate from grains and vegetables. As a result, it might be necessary to change the balance or nature of carbohydrate intake by increasing, reducing or changing sources in the diet to improve overall balance. Detailed suggestions for actual foods to add or reduce in the diet could be obtained from listings of individual foods that are easily available in textbooks or on the internet.

This same approach could be used to then address any imbalance in protein intake by considering the current balance between animal (eg. meat, fish, dairy) and plant (eg. legumes, nuts, seeds, pulses, soya) sources. Again, more detailed food lists would give ideas of protein foods to add or reduce in the diet. Similarly, food lists could be used to identify additional dietary sources of vitamin D if this vitamin is needed. This approach can be repeated for all the food groups noted in the checklists, and the checklists themselves could be re-designed as required to suit those using them.

Any actions identified can be grouped together by nutrition professionals planning consultations, or allocated to different weeks/months by an individual working alone, to create a plan of interventions over time. Each completed or planned change can be ticked, and/or highlighted in a range of colours, and/or dated on the chart to track progress. The sheets can be printed and kept by a nutrition professional in the patient's notes, or by an individual in a suitable file.

Table 4.1: Food addiction: nutritional approaches checklist

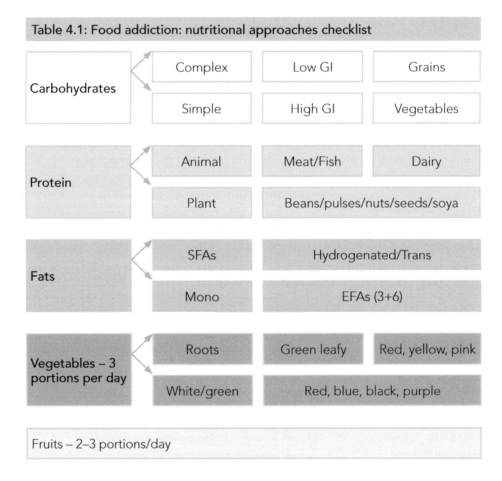

| Carbohydrates | Complex | Low GI | Grains |
| | Simple | High GI | Vegetables |

| Protein | Animal | Meat/Fish | Dairy |
| | Plant | Beans/pulses/nuts/seeds/soya | |

| Fats | SFAs | Hydrogenated/Trans | |
| | Mono | EFAs (3+6) | |

| Vegetables – 3 portions per day | Roots | Green leafy | Red, yellow, pink |
| | White/green | Red, blue, black, purple | |

Fruits – 2–3 portions/day

Table 4.2: Food addiction: nutritional approaches checklist

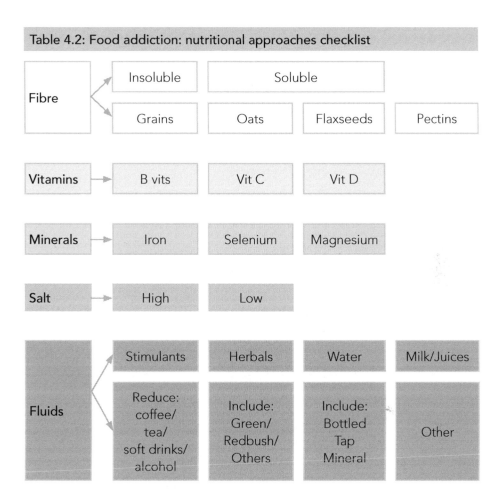

Fibre	Insoluble	Soluble		
	Grains	Oats	Flaxseeds	Pectins

Vitamins	B vits	Vit C	Vit D

Minerals	Iron	Selenium	Magnesium

Salt	High	Low

Fluids	Stimulants	Herbals	Water	Milk/Juices
	Reduce: coffee/ tea/ soft drinks/ alcohol	Include: Green/ Redbush/ Others	Include: Bottled Tap Mineral	Other

Chapter 5

Chocolate addiction

Ann Woodriff Beirne

Introduction

Chocolate – food of the gods and a sweet temptation to many who claim they are 'addicted' to it. But is it possible to be addicted to chocolate? It is generally thought that the answer is no as the chemicals in chocolate are either not chemically addictive, or not present in sufficient quantities to account for an addiction. Yet there are many people who have difficulty cutting it out of their diet, or even reducing it to a small amount that is eaten occasionally.

Why is chocolate so tempting? Does it really contain chemically-addictive components in sufficient quantities to cause an actual physical addiction? Or is it more a psychological addiction that depends on the comforting qualities of the organoleptic experience of taste and mouthfeel? This chapter explores some of the myths and truths about chocolate, and our relationship with it.

Chocolate consumption worldwide

Graph 5.1 shows the highest world consumers of chocolate in terms of average kilograms per head of population. Considering that some people will eat far less than the average amount, it is likely that others will make up the difference by eating far more.

There is no breakdown available in the figures between dark chocolate and milk chocolate, which is regrettable as there is a big difference between the two types in terms of chemical content, sugar and fat content and health implications. White chocolate is also included in these figures, however, white chocolate contains no cocoa solids, only cocoa butter, and therefore contains none of the chemicals of interest, nor does it have any of the health benefits. It also has the highest sugar and fat content, and it is debatable whether it even deserves the name 'chocolate'.

The graph shows countries with the highest chocolate consumption per person in 2005, compared to the figures from 2002. [1]

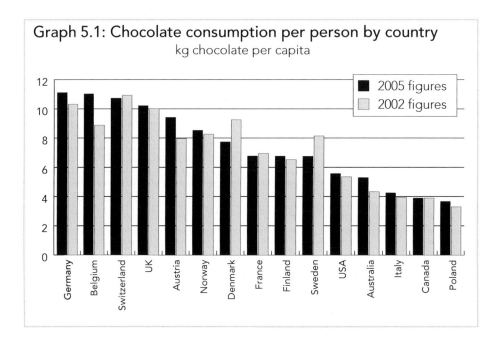

Graph 5.1: Chocolate consumption per person by country
kg chocolate per capita

Brief history of chocolate

Chocolate first came to the attention of the western world when the Spanish conquistadors brought it back with them after their forays into Central and South America. The word 'cacao' comes from the language of the Mayan people who were the earliest users of the cacao bean. The word 'chocolate' is derived from the Aztec word *'cacahuatl'*. In both Mayan and Aztec cultures, chocolate had divine origins. It was given to the people by the gods (the Mayan god, Ek Chuah and the Aztec god, Quetzalcoatl) and was frequently used as an offering in many rituals. In these cultures

1   Workman D (2007) *Chocolate Covered Countries: US sales of premium dark and gourmet chocolate gifts soar* [online]. Available at: http://www.suite101.com/content/chocolate-covered-countries-a26240 (accessed August 2011).

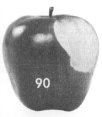

chocolate was served as a beverage to only high-ranking adult males and sacrifice victims. The beverage contained spices – notably chilli – and while not being very sweet, it was considered powerful and intoxicating and therefore unsuitable for women and children.

The cocoa bean was an expensive commodity and commanded a high trade price. The Spanish introduced it to Europe, initially as a drink, and it took off rapidly around much of the rest of western Europe where it was valued both for its culinary and medicinal properties.

Solid chocolate was first created by Joseph Fry in 1847. Since then, chocolate manufacture has become big business, made so by people's desire for the sweet, seductive taste of the confection.

What drives the desire?

As stated, both the Aztecs and Mayans believed that their chocolate beverage had intoxicating and strengthening powers. Montezuma, emperor of the Aztecs, always took a cup of chocolate before visiting his wives as he believed it was also an aphrodisiac. But what is it about chocolate that attracts people so much?

Chemical factors

Chocolate contains a number of chemicals – mainly alkaloids which are compounds produced by plants that can have potent effects – and they have the ability to trigger physiological reactions in the body. These are caffeine, theobromine, phenylethylamine (PEA) and anandamide. Current research suggests that the levels of these chemicals in an average bar of chocolate are insufficient to cause any real physiological effects, so the case for them triggering a full chemical addiction is poor. To test this, a group of researchers created a drink and gave it to two groups of test subjects. One group was also given a capsule containing 19mg caffeine and 250mg theobromine, similar to the amounts found in a 100g bar of milk chocolate; and the other group was given a placebo. Subjective responses for liking the drink and various taste and sensory descriptors showed a significant increase in the group given the caffeine and theobromine capsule over the placebo group, leading the researchers to conclude that the caffeine and theobromine *'may well contribute to the liking for chocolate, especially in the more acquired taste for dark chocolate'.*[2]

Research performed in 1994, on the other hand, suggests that there is little chance of any pharmacological effect. A group of self-confessed chocolate addicts were divided into five groups. At the start of the craving the groups were each given a box containing one of the following:

1. milk chocolate bar

2. white chocolate bar (no pharmacological agents that are present in cacao)

3. cocoa capsules

4. placebo

5. nothing.

The milk chocolate and white chocolate both reduced chocolate cravings, although the white chocolate only did so partially, while the cocoa capsules (containing all the psychopharmacological agents) did not. This suggests that the organoleptic properties of chocolate are the main reasons for the craving, at least in the individuals tested.[3]

Another argument against these substances causing a chemical addiction is the fact that milk chocolate is still preferred by many 'addicts'. Milk chocolate contains even less of the active substances than cocoa-rich dark chocolate and also contains higher levels of sugar and fat. It has been suggested, therefore, that it is sugar that creates the desire. Yet, if you were to offer people the same amount of sugar as found in their chocolate bar they would not be tempted in by it in the same way.

Organoleptic factors

It could be the combination of sugar and fat ie. the 'mouthfeel' or organoleptic experience that makes people crave chocolate. Cocoa butter has a melting point of around 34–38⁰C, which is perfect for melting in the mouth and giving that luxurious sensation of molten chocolate. But a simple experiment with the herb Gymnema silvestre shows that mouthfeel is not the full answer

2   Smit HJ & Blackburn RJ (2005) Reinforcing effects of caffeine and theobromine as found in chocolate. *Psychopharmacology* **181** (1) 101–106.

3   Michener W & Rozin P (1994) Pharmacological versus sensory factors in the satiation of chocolate craving. *Physiology & Behaviour* **56** (3) 419–422.

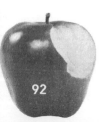

either – Gymnema blocks the sweetness receptors on the tongue temporarily so that you cannot taste sweetness. Eating chocolate after consuming some Gymnema is distressing for the chocolate-lover as it does not taste sweet – in fact it tastes more like mud. All you experience is a fatty substance melting in your mouth, and it is not too pleasant.

So is it just the taste itself then? Or the aroma? Chocolate, along with coffee and roast beef, has been shown to have a high impact on saliva induction in test subjects – smelling these items induces a 'want to eat' response.

Is it the combination of all of the above? According to subjective testing, it is indeed likely to be the entire combination: the taste, aroma, mouthfeel and sweetness.

Other factors

Another potential area for research is in neurobiology; live imaging (eg. functional magnetic resonance imaging, or fMRI) can show which parts of the brain respond to various stimuli, including the pleasure response from eating chocolate.

Some research has suggested that women are more prone to chocolate 'addiction' than men and that this may be, in part, related to women's fluctuating hormones. But then, it has also been suggested that eating chocolate is a response to the body requiring extra minerals such as magnesium. Chocolate may be a source of magnesium, but so are dark green leafy vegetables and most people do not experience the same cravings for spinach or Brussels sprouts.

There is also the conditioning aspect to consider. Advertising has frequently associated chocolate with love and romance – the Milk Tray advert, for example – or with self-indulgence – the Cadbury's Flake adverts from the 1980s, and the later Galaxy adverts as other examples, which reinforces mental images of chocolate in these settings.

Other factors such as hunger, mood or mental state can also influence individual responses to chocolate.

The chemicals in chocolate that may be addictive

As mentioned above, the chemicals found in chocolate include caffeine, theobromine, phenylethylamine and anandamide. Caffeine is the most well known of these and is also found in coffee, tea and cola drinks.

Caffeine

The media frequently reports that there is much less caffeine in chocolate than in a cup of coffee. This is a nonsensical statement as the amount of caffeine in a cup of coffee varies enormously, depending on the type of coffee, the size of the cup (see Table 5.1), the brand and personal preference for strength. It also depends on what type of chocolate is being referred to – a high cocoa-solids chocolate contains more caffeine than a bar of milk chocolate – so comparing chocolate and a cup of coffee is futile.

Due to the variations between manufacturers, the figures in Table 5.1 are approximations. However, it does show that there is more caffeine in 100g of dark chocolate than there is in a single cup of most instant coffees and many filtered coffees.

The effects of caffeine in the body

Caffeine has stimulant effects on the nervous system; it causes adrenalin to be released by the nerve cells and this can affect blood sugar levels, raise the heart rate, blood pressure and blood flow to the muscles (the 'fight or flight' effect).

Table 5.1				
	Quantity		Caffeine content	
Substance	US measure	Metric	Mg	mg/ 100ml or 100g
Double espresso	2oz	59ml	58–185	98–313
Single espresso	2oz	59ml	29–100	49–169
Drip-filtered coffee	6oz	177ml	80–200	45–113
Black tea	7oz	207ml	58–86	28–41.5
Instant coffee	8oz	237ml	65–90*	28–38
White tea	7oz	207ml	56–75	27.1–36.2

Table 5.1 (continued)				
Red Bull	8.4oz	248ml	80	32.2
Pepsi Max	8oz	237ml	69	29.2
Green tea	7oz	207ml	59	28.5
Pepsi Cola	8oz	237ml	38	16.1
Coca Cola	8oz	237ml	34	14.4
Diet Coke	8oz	237ml	30	12.7
SlimFast chocolate drink	1 serve	325ml	20	6.2
Chocolate milk	8oz	237ml	4	1.7
Dark chocolate	**1oz**	**28g**	**20**	**71.4**
Milk chocolate	**1oz**	**28g**	**6**	**21.4**
* most common range, although it can vary from 27–273mg in an 8oz cup (11–115mg/100ml)				

Figures taken from http://coffeetea.about.com/library/blcaffeine.htm[4]

Caffeine is also a mild diuretic and a psychoactive compound ie. it has the ability to affect mood, perceptions and emotions. Although caffeine is quickly removed from the brain, thus having only short-term effects, people can build up tolerance to it, leading them to need more and more to achieve the same effects. If caffeine is removed from the diet, withdrawal symptoms are commonly mild to severe headaches, which may last for a few days; feelings of depression; and sleepiness. Caffeine withdrawal is a recognised condition that may affect people's ability to function properly. Caffeine can therefore be considered as an addictive component of chocolate.

Theobromine

The level of theobromine in chocolate and cocoa is widely variable, reportedly from 10mg/g in dark chocolate, 1–5 mg/g in milk chocolate and 11–43mg/g in cocoa beans. Theobromine is chemically related to caffeine, but has much milder effects and is found in higher (but variably so) quantities than caffeine in chocolate and cocoa products.

The effects of theobromine in the body

Theobromine relaxes the smooth muscles of the bronchi, is a mild stimulant and a mild diuretic. It causes blood vessels to relax and therefore can be used to reduce blood pressure (this may be a natural counter measure

---

4   Goodwin L (2011) How much caffeine is in coffee, tea, cola and other drinks? [online] Available at: http://coffeetea.about.com/library/blcaffeine.htm (accessed August 2011).

against the effects of the caffeine). Although theobromine is less stimulating in nature than caffeine, it has a higher capacity to improve mood and is well absorbed from chocolate (about 80% of the absorption of theobromine in solution).[5] Theobromine has toxic effects on the heart, central nervous system and kidneys in dogs. This is why dogs should not be given chocolate that is made for human consumption.

Phenylethylamine

Phenylethylamine (PEA) is a substance found in chocolate that is also created by our bodies as a natural mood enhancer.

The effects of phenylethylamine in the body

PEA is distributed throughout the central nervous system and produced naturally by brain tissue. It is dopaminergic ie. it stimulates the production of dopamine, which is an important neurotransmitter. This can lead the nervous system to produce feelings similar to when one is 'in love' by stimulating the brain's pleasure/reward centres, which is why chocolate has been said to possess aphrodisiac qualities (considered mythical by many). Its effects on mood include the ability to increase attention and activity in animals and relieve depression in 60% of depressed patients when given orally in doses of 10–60mg per day. The results were as rapid as those achieved with amphetamines but with no tolerance induction (ie. the participants didn't need ever increasing dosages to achieve the same effect).[6]

As an important mood modulator, PEA has been a prime candidate for the chemical in chocolate that causes us to reach for it when we feel down and depressed. Scientists have suggested that low levels of PEA in the body are a contributing factor for low mood, so it would make sense for us to try to obtain PEA from elsewhere. However, the enzyme monoamine oxidase B (MAO-B) breaks down PEA and other scientists maintain that any PEA we take in via chocolate would not reach our brain receptors because it would be broken down in the gut.

A breakdown product of PEA is a substance called phenylacetic acid (PAA), which is found in urine. PAA levels have been shown to be lower in depressed and bipolar patients than in the normal healthy population, to the extent

5   Shively CA, Tarka SM Jr, Arnaud MJ, Dvorchik BH, Passananti GT & Vesell ES (1985) High levels of methylxanthines in chocolate do not alter theobromine disposition. *Clinical Pharmacology and Therapeutics* **37** (4) 415–424.

6   Sabelli H, Fink P, Fawcett J & Tom C (1996) Sustained antidepressant effect of PEA replacement. *Journal of Neuropsychiatry and Clinical Neuroscience* **8** (2) 168–171.

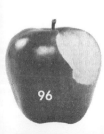

that low levels of urinary and plasma PAA are considered a marker for depression. L-phenylalanine, a precursor to PEA, has also been shown to enhance mood in some depressed patients, who subsequently show an increase in urinary PAA. Although L-phenylalanine is also a precursor to catecholamine neurotransmitters, it appears that it is being used in the body to make PEA, which is then broken down to PAA and excreted in the urine.[7]

One class of antidepressant drugs are the monoamine oxidase inhibitors (MAOIs). If a person is taking these drugs to slow down the breakdown of natural PEA in the body, then any PEA eaten in the form of chocolate would also last longer and is less likely to be broken down, so it is possible that PEA from chocolate has a contributory positive effect on mood in depressed patients on MAOI drugs.

As well as working on PEA, MAOIs affect the breakdown of tyramine (an amino acid found in various foods). High levels of tyramine in the body can result in raised blood pressure and migraines, so patients taking MAOIs are advised to strictly limit their intake of tyramine-containing foods because of the risk. If MAOIs are limiting the breakdown of tyramines to the extent that they could cause harm, it is a reasonable assumption that they inhibit the breakdown of PEA sufficiently to allow it to have an effect on mood as well. However, there is, as yet, no scientific evidence to show that PEA specifically from chocolate lasts long enough in the body to trigger the pleasure centres in the brain.

Anandamide

Anandamide is another neurochemical made in the body. It was discovered in 1992 and is known as the bliss molecule (from the Sanskrit word for 'bliss'). It is part of the endocannabinoid system, which is named after the THC (tetrahydrocannabinol) receptor in the brain. The THC receptor is activated by, among other substances, cannabinols found in Sativa cannabis, the cannabis plant. When people take in large quantities of cannabinols from this plant, THC receptors in the brain are activated, thus engendering a 'feel-good' state. Endocannabinoids are chemicals that we produce ourselves that are similar to these cannabinols and also trigger the THC receptor.

---

7   Sabelli HC, Fawcett J, Gusovsky F, Javaid JI, Wynn P, Edwards J, Jeffriess H & Kravitz H (1986) Clinical studies on the phenylethylamine hypothesis of affective disorder: urine and blood phenylacetic acid and phenylalanine dietary supplements. *Journal of Clinical Psychiatry* **47** (2) 66–70.

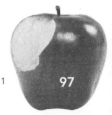

The amount of anandamide (or anandamide-like substances) in chocolate is not the highest in any food; there are other foods which contain more anandamide (such as salami or some cheeses), but there may be a synergistic effect with the other alkaloids in chocolate, giving a larger response than is achievable with anandamide alone. Chocolate also contains N-acylethanolamines which block the breakdown of anandamide. Despite all this, the effect of anandamide on the THC receptors is minuscule in comparison with cannabis.

The effects of anandamide in the body

Anandamide attaches to and activates the THC receptors in the brain, producing a feeling of well-being; when these THC receptors are activated in excess, it gives rise to the person feeling 'blissed out'. The brain uses enzymes such as monoamine oxidase to break down anandamide rapidly to prevent over activation of the brain (refer to section on PEA regarding the use of MAOIs) – so not only does taking MAOIs inhibit the breakdown of PEA, there will also be a reduction in breakdown of anandamide.

Research has shown that chocolate contains not only a small amount of anandamide, but also two similar molecules, N-oleoylethanolamine and N-linoleoylethanolamine.[8] These compounds were shown in cell culture to inhibit the breakdown of anandamide, thus potentially prolonging the 'bliss' effect.[9] However, it has not been established whether there are sufficient quantities of any of these substances in chocolate, or whether they would even reach the brain to have any effect.

On testing anandamide passage through the digestive tract of rats, it appears that digestive enzymes limit the absorption of anandamide[10] and that to achieve a psychotropic effect, much higher doses than could be found in chocolate would be required. However, the presence or effect of the two ethanolamines present in chocolate that have the potential to inhibit anandamide breakdown were not tested for.

Anandamide is therefore another prime contender for the reason why people crave chocolate when they feel depressed, miserable or need a bit of comfort food. It has been suggested, however, that chocolate contains so little anandamide that a person would need to consume several kilos of chocolate

8   Di Tomasso E, Beltramo M & Pomelli D (1996) Brain cannabinoids in chocolate. *Nature* **382** 677–678.

9   Pomelli D (1996) Interview with Normal Swan on ABC Radio – Health Report [online]. Available at: http://www.abc.net.au/rn/talks/8.30/helthrpt/hstories/hr260896.htm (accessed August 2011).

10   Di Marzo V, Sepe N, De Petrocellis L, Berger A, Crozier G, Fride E & Mechoulam R (1998) Trick or treat from food cannabinoids? *Nature* **396** 636–637.

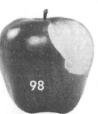

(11kg for a person weighing 130lb[11]) in one sitting to achieve any noticeable biochemical effect. So far, the research suggests it would be physically impossible to eat enough chocolate to trigger THC receptors to the same extent that cannabis does – one would be 'sick of it' before any 'high' was reached.

Other alkaloids

Another psychoactive, dopaminergic alkaloid found in chocolate is salsolinol. It has been found at concentrations of up to 25ug/g – potentially active levels in humans.[12] Tetrahydro-beta carbolines are also present in chocolate. These are compounds found in alcoholic drinks, which have been linked to alcoholism. It is possible that they inhibit MAO and thus may increase or prolong the effects of PEA and anandamide.[6]

Box 5.1: Why chocolate?
We like chocolate because we are programmed genetically to like sweet/ fat combinations that taste extremely good. When we eat something we like, we produce endorphins. This is not exclusive to chocolate – anything that tastes good induces brain endorphin release. Professor David Benton (Department Psychology, University of Wales – 1998 Kellogg Nutrition Symposium in Sydney)

Organoleptic factors

Fat and sugar
Fat and sugar together produce a highly palatable combination. The sugar provides the sweetness that we crave, while the fat contributes a silky smoothness that feels good in the mouth. Buttercream icing is a classic example of how good this combination can be for sweet-toothed individuals.

According to Drewnowski *et al* (1992), the effects of eating highly palatable foods, ie. those high in sugar and fat such as chocolate, can stimulate the production of endogenous opioids (opiate-like substances), also known as endorphins. In a test situation, 14 female binge eaters (eight of whom were obese) and 12 normal controls were given naloxone, an opioid antagonist

11 Kuwana E (2010) Discovering the sweet mysteries of chocolate [online]. Available at: http://faculty. washington.edu/chudler/choco.html (accessed August 2011).

12 Melzig MF, Putscher I, Henklein P & Haber H (2000) In vitro pharmacological activity of the tetrahydroisoquinoline salsolinol present in products from Theobroma cacao L. like cocoa and chocolate. *Journal of Ethnopharmacology* **73** 153–159.

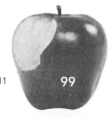

drug, which not only reduced caloric intake of sweet fatty foods in binge eaters, it seemed to reduce the preference for such foods in all test subjects (binge eaters and normal controls). This suggests endorphins may be involved in mediating taste preferences for high fat/sugar foods.[13]

This same research group also suggested sweet cravings may be associated with opiate addiction and that withdrawal from opiates may be eased by eating sweets. This hypothesis ties in with dopamine research on obese individuals and drug addicts that shows their altered dopamine responses and enhanced need for the addictive behaviour of choice.

A questionnaire on the behaviour of 50 self-confessed chocoholics demonstrated that 75% defined their 'addiction' by how the chocolate tasted and felt, and also by their own lack of control.[14] Many experienced negative feelings after eating chocolate (eg. self-loathing and guilt), which would often result in a cyclic pattern of eating more to feel better, then feeling bad again. Out of the 50 who were questioned, only five preferred dark chocolate, indicating again that the organoleptic features of chocolate are more likely to be involved in chocolate 'addiction' than the psychopharmacological agents that are present in much lower quantities in the preferred milk chocolate.

The fat and sugar percentage/ratio seems to make little difference when it comes to 'addiction'. As has been already stated with the cocoa content, fat and sugar content *and* ratio varies between manufacturers, and between dark, milk and white chocolates. There is not a single standard ratio of fat to sugar within chocolate. Connoisseurs of chocolate are just as able to tell one brand from the other as wine-tasting experts. Although this may have something to do with the roasting and manufacturing process, as well as the type(s) of cacao bean in use, it will also be linked to the quantities of the macronutrients fat and sugar.

Leptin is a regulatory peptide in the homeostatic control of appetite. It provides negative feedback and is produced as we become full, inhibiting our feelings of hunger. High serum leptin levels have been associated with lower intake of, and reduced preference for, high fat/high sugar foods in

13   Drewnoski A, Krahn DD, Demitrack MA, Nairn K & Gosnell BA (1992) Taste responses and preferences for sweet high-fat foods: evidence for opioid involvement. *Physiology and Behaviour* **51** (2) 371–379.

14   Hetherington MM & MacDiarmid JI (1993) Chocolate addiction: a preliminary study of its description and its relationship to problem eating. *Appetite* **21** (3) 233–246.

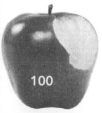

obese women.[15] Larsson *et al* reported that higher levels of serum leptin reduced caloric intake overall and also reduced carbohydrate and saturated fat intake in post-menopausal women of varying body shape and body fat.[16]

Other factors

Neurobiological responses
Dopamine response
As has been noted, most of the potentially psychoactive components of chocolate are dopaminergic in nature ie. they promote the production of dopamine. Research into the dopamine response in addictive behaviours has thrown up some interesting discoveries.

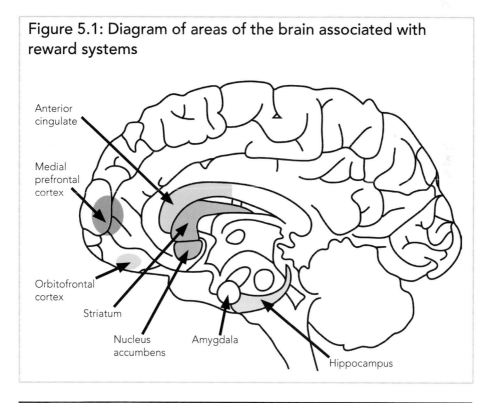

Figure 5.1: Diagram of areas of the brain associated with reward systems

15   Karhunen LJ, Lappalainen RI, Haffner SM, Valve RH, Tuorila H, Miettinen H & Uusitupa MI (1998) Serum leptin, food intake and preferences for sugar and fat in obese women. *International Journal of Obesity Relaed Metabolic Disorders* **22** (8) 819–821.

16   Larsson H, Elmstahl S, Berglund G & Ahren B (1998) Evidence for leptin regulation of food intake in humans. *Journal of Clinical Endocrinology and Metabolism* **83** (12) 4382–4385.

It is known that substances of abuse, drugs and alcohol also activate a dopamine response, specifically the dopaminergic mesolimbic reinforcement system, or 'reward system'. The dopamine that is produced is released to the nucleus accumbens (NAC) in the brain, which may cause the hedonistic response to incentives. It has been known for at least 10 years that food can also cause a short-term release of dopamine to the NAC. The need to eat food is triggered primarily by the homeostatic regulation of appetite, in other words, being hungry and then feeling full after eating, but it has become apparent through neuroendocrine and brain imaging studies that the motivation and reward systems also play a part in initiating eating.[17]

This has led to a potential link between obesity and other addictive disorders. In people with addictive disorders, there may be adaptive processes within the reward system that reinforce the addictive behaviour. Negative outcomes do not provide sufficient impact; they are not 'learnt' and therefore the addictive behaviour is unchecked. High fat/high carbohydrate foods in particular appear to act as reinforcers for impulsive, addictive behaviour, in a similar way to addictive drugs.[17]

The appetite regulating peptides, leptin, ghrelin and orexin have been shown to modulate the dopaminergic response, thus providing a link between the homeostatic control of appetite and the mesolimbic reward system.[17] High levels of leptin and low levels of ghrelin and orexin cause a reduction in dopamine, which in turn leads to cravings for the substances that will boost the dopamine reward system.

Leptin: High levels of leptin provide negative feedback and reduce appetite. High levels of leptin also lead to reduced extracellular dopamine and have been shown to correlate with increased alcohol intake in alcoholic subjects. Reduced dopaminergic activity at least partially increases the reward effect of addictive substances.

Ghrelin: Stimulates appetite, food intake and weight gain. Ghrelin also stimulates dopamine release in the NAC. Ghrelin receptor dysfunction and antagonism can lead to reduced intake of addictive substances. Alcoholics show increased plasma ghrelin levels.

Orexin (hypocretin): This is activated by hypoglycaemia and other appetite-associated peptides (such as ghrelin) and leads to increased appetite.

---

17   Grosshans M, Loeber S, & Kiefer F (2011) Implications from addiction research towards the understanding and treatment of obesity. *Addiction Biology* **16** 189–198.

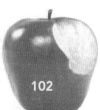

Hyperglycaemia and leptin inhibit orexin secretion. Orexin stimulates dopamine release in the NAC. Orexin-receptor antagonists reduce alcohol resumption in alcoholic rats, and reduce reward-based feeding.[17]

As there is this association between obesity and substance addiction, it has been suggested that obesity should be recognised as a mental disorder in the forthcoming DSM-V. As already stated, some foods may trigger the release of dopamine to the NAC – a direct function of the palatability and reward levels of the food – chocolate being extremely palatable and rewarding for most people. This function of food can be associated or dissociated from the homeostatic regulation of food intake (hunger/satiety) – in other words, if you are hungry you are more likely to want to eat something nice than not; but even if you are not hungry you might still want to eat something nice and rewarding, like chocolate.[18]

The endocannabinoid and opioid reward systems are also relevant to food ingestion – and as we have seen, some components of chocolate have the potential to trigger both of these.

The reinforcing effects of psychostimulant drugs correlate with increased brain dopamine levels and the subjective perception of reward/pleasure[18] – the same appears to be true of chocolate consumption. Increased regional blood flow to the dorsal striatum has been demonstrated during the ingestion of chocolate and a positive correlation between blood flow and the sensation of pleasure from its consumption. Drug 'reward' is processed more by the ventral striatum, so there is a slight distinction between the reward processing of food and drugs, but still an overlap. In a study comparing chocolate cravers to non-cravers, cravers showed greater activation in reward areas (medial prefrontal cortex, anterior cingulate and ventral striatum), many of which overlap with those activated in drug craving studies. However, in drug craving studies, drug addicts were used, whereas normal healthy individuals were used in the chocolate craving studies (rather than obese individuals). There may be a different pattern in obese people, as studies are showing their responses to foods can differ from healthy-weighted people.[18]

It is possible that when the food reward system is dysfunctional, it is involved in the move towards obesity. When tested, obese people (BMI

---

18   Frascella J, Potenza MN, Brown L & Childress AR (2010) Shared brain vulnerabilities open the way for non-substance addictions: carving addiction at a new joint? *Annals of the New York Academy of Science* **1187** 294–315.

between 42 and 60) have been found to have fewer D2-dopamine receptors, particularly striatal dopamine receptors. Dorsal striatal receptors are activated selectively by high fat, high carbohydrate foods and produce a significantly greater motivational emotional response in obese women; and reduction in D2 receptor levels has been linked to decreased sensitivity to the consequences of negative actions [18] (eg. realising that eating more is associated with weight gain).

A possible genetic link with the A1 allele of the Taq1 gene and underfunctioning of the dorsal striatum has been found in people with addictive behaviours, including overeating. There is an association between higher BMI and presence of this gene allele.[18]

Serotonin response[19]

The neurotransmitter serotonin has also been put forward as a contributor to the 'addictive' effects of chocolate. Serotonin, or 5-hydroxytryptamine (5-HT), is another endorphin that we produce ourselves, derived from the amino acid tryptophan; it is linked to appetite, impulse control and mood elevation. A lack of serotonin is a known cause of depression and it has been suggested that carbohydrate/chocolate consumption may be a form of 'self-medication' to address this.

The proposed mechanism suggests that as carbohydrates stimulate insulin production, this facilitates the uptake of amino acids (except tryptophan) into the tissues, leaving a relatively high ratio of circulating tryptophan, which can then more easily pass across the blood–brain barrier and be converted to serotonin. However, the relationship between depression and appetite is more complex than first appears; not all depressive patients find eating helps, in fact many lose their appetite. Another flaw in this hypothesis is that the protein component of the food needs to be less than 2% to favour an increase in brain serotonin levels; chocolate typically contains 3–22% protein.[20] Further, changes in tryptophan levels are too slow to account for the immediate mood lift post-consumption; and these mood improvements can happen without any concomitant change in serotonin synthesis and release. It is therefore unlikely that serotonin levels are directly linked to the mood improvements experienced by some after chocolate consumption.

19   Parker G, Parker I & Brotchie H (2006) Mood state effects of chocolate. *Journal of Affective Disorders* **92** (2–3)149–159.

20   Cacao Web (2011) Nutrition facts for cocoa and chocolate [online]. Available at: http://www.cacaoweb.net/nutrition.html (accessed August 2011).

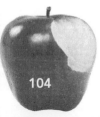

Opioid response to casomorphins

There is some evidence that inefficient digestion of milk products may produce opioid-like substances called casomorphins. Researchers speculate that where there is a 'leaky gut' situation, casomorphins reach the opioid receptors in the brain, triggering the opioid reward system. In this particular set of circumstances, more reward would be gained from higher milk content – so milk chocolate and white chocolate would be the chocolates of choice. However, if this were the only modality causing an 'addiction' to chocolate, then there would be other sources of milk/milk products that could provide a better casomorphin 'hit' than milk chocolate.

Hormones

A research group tested for chocolate liking/craving among 249 students and 319 of their parents.[21] The results showed that:

■ more females had cravings, especially during their perimenstrual time

■ there was no significant correlation between parents and children liking chocolate, so a genetic link appeared unlikely

■ sensory appeal was the primary motivator

■ there was little evidence for any pharmacological influence on the liking for chocolate, based on correlational data from the study.

Some studies have suggested that cravings for chocolate are higher among females and it appears that cravings increase with premenstrual syndrome (PMS). There may be a physiological link in that chocolate is a source of magnesium, and low levels of magnesium have been identified in women with PMS.

However, it may be psychological – the range of symptoms that can accompany PMS include bloating, lower back pain, spots, sensitive breasts, tearfulness, irritability and mood swings. This may impact on the woman's feelings of attractiveness and eating chocolate may allow them to enter the fantasy world of feeling loved that they have been conditioned to respond to by advertising.

---

21   Rozin P, Levine E & Stoess C (1991) Chocolate craving and liking. *Appetite* **17** (3) 199–212.

Mood

Emotions can affect chocolate consumption and enjoyment. There is a general perception that chocolate is a 'comfort food' and that people eat it when they are sad, but this was not the experience of one researcher, who discovered that healthy males consumed less chocolate when sadness was induced in them than when happiness was; the happy state increased both consumption and enjoyment of the chocolate.[22] This experiment was conducted on men – it may have shown different results with women. It also highlights different modalities; emotional-congruent eating (demonstrated in this experiment) as opposed to eating in order to regulate emotions (the so-called 'comfort eating').

Another researcher asked 20 self-confessed 'addicts' and 20 non-addicts to keep a diary for two days, during which they rated feelings of depression, anxiety, guilt, craving, relaxation and contentment both before and after eating chocolate. The results showed that the addicts had higher rates of negative and lower positive feelings before eating chocolate, but that their positive feelings did not significantly improve after consumption; rather their feelings of guilt increased, especially if the chocolate intake was excessive in their eyes.[23] So 'comfort eating' for an 'addict' appears to be an incorrect perception – at least in this small study. The addicts also showed higher indications of disordered eating patterns.

This last finding was replicated by another researcher who reported a significant relationship between chocolate 'addiction' and aberrant eating behaviours; and also that the 'addicts' had significantly higher rates of depression than the controls.[24]

On the other hand, Dallard *et al* (2001) concluded that the 15 chocoholics he tested *do not seem to suffer from eating disorders but may represent a population of psychologically vulnerable and depression or anxiety-prone people. They seem to use chocolate as a light psychotropic drug able to relieve some of their distress ... and they rarely display other addictive*

---

22   Macht M, Roth S & Ellgring H (2002) Chocolate eating in healthy men during experimentally induced sadness and joy. *Appetite* **39** (2) 147–158.

23   Macdiarmid JI & Hetherington MM (1995) Mood modulation by food: an exploration of affect and cravings in 'chocolate addicts'. *British Journal of Clinical Psychology* **34** (1) 129–138.

24   Tuomisto T, Hetherington MM, Morris MF, Tuomisto MT, Turjanmaa V & Lappalainen R (1999) Psychological and physiological characteristics of sweet food "addiction". *International Journal of Eating Disorders* **25** (2) 169–167.

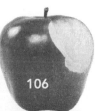

behaviours.[25] Although none of Dallard *et al's* subjects registered on the eating disorder scales, 13 of them had a history of major depressive episodes and four had anxiety disorders.[25]

In 2004 Smit *et al* did some research on the cognitive performance and mood change induced by chocolate. They tested subjects with three types of chocolate (dark, milk and white), cocoa powder and a caffeine and theobromine mixture, using water as the placebo. Both the cocoa powder and the caffeine/theobromine mix showed improvements in cognitive function and increased perception of energy, versus water; and the milk and dark chocolate both showed significant improvements in cognitive function compared with white chocolate. From this, the researchers deduced that the methylxanthines (caffeine and theobromine) in chocolate have the ability to produce psychopharmacological activity in humans.[26]

A group of researchers at Swansea University played sad films to students to depress their moods. They discovered that as the students' mood decreased, their need for chocolate rose. Half of the students were given chocolate and the other half were given carob, a chocolate substitute. The half given chocolate experienced an uplift in mood, whereas those given carob did not.[27]

Hunger

Eating chocolate when hungry may increase the craving for it, as shown by a study carried out on both chocolate cravers and non-cravers. Each group was divided in half, and each half was given chocolate to eat twice a day for 14 days. However, one half of the group was asked to eat their chocolate 15–30 minutes after eating a full meal; the other half was asked to wait two hours after eating a full meal before consuming the chocolate. Each participant kept a diary and recorded daily the amount of chocolate consumed, the anticipatory pleasure ratings and the actual pleasure rating on eating the chocolate. The ones who ate chocolate while full from their meal found they had decreased chocolate cravings, regardless of whether or not they were hungry; whereas those who ate chocolate after their

25   Dallard I, Cathebras P, Sauron C & Massoubre C (2001) Is cocoa a psychotropic drug? Psychopathologic study of a population of subjects self-identified as chocolate addicts. *Encephale* **27** (2) 181–186.
26   Smit HJ, Gaffan EA & Rogers PJ (2004) Methylxanthines are the psycho-pharmacologically active constituents of chocolate. *Psychopharmacology* **176** (3–4) 412–419.
27   Willner P, Benton D, Brown E, Cheeta S, Davies G, Morgan J & Morgan M (1998) "Depression" increases "craving" for sweet rewards in animal and human models of depression and craving. *Psychopharmacology (Berlin)* **136** (3) 272–283.

fullness had dissipated found that their cravings increased.[28] This points to a learned appetite response involvement in the craving, which offers the potential to be altered to reduce the craving.

Research on brain responses to eating chocolate past the point of satiety has shown that different areas of the brain respond according to whether eating chocolate is still pleasurable or not[29] and that men and women have different brain responses when eating chocolate beyond their comfort point.[30] The orbito-frontal cortex (OFC) response was especially noted; while pleasure was still the outcome, the caudomedial part of the OFC responded, suggesting that it is associated with the pleasure response. However, when it no longer became pleasurable to eat the chocolate, the caudolateral OFC responded instead,[29] suggesting it to be an area associated with avoidance behaviours.

Socio-cultural effects

It has been suggested that much of chocolate addiction may be due to social conditioning.[31] In other words, the general perception, perpetuated by the media, is that chocolate is a treat (often forbidden), an indulgence, and something that people may feel the need to hide from others. However, family interactions may also contribute to this; grandparents often covertly indulge their grandchildren with chocolate and sweets, far more than their parents would allow, thus adding to the brain pathways associating chocolate with love and secrecy.

Restricting chocolate tends to increase the desire for it, especially if one tries to stop before satiety, leading to the idea of 'moreishness', craving, and, in more extreme cases, 'addiction'.

Interestingly, one research group who tested the differences in chocolate cravings between Spanish and American populations discovered that in America the rates of self-confessed 'addicts' was 91% of females and 59% of males; whereas in the Spanish population the male rate increased to 78%

28   Gibson EL & Desmond E (1999) Chocolate craving and hunger state: implications for the acquisition and expression of appetite and food choice. *Appetite* **32** (2) 219–240.

29   Small DM, Zatorre RJ, Dagher A, Evans AC & Jones-Gotman M (2001) Changes in brain activity related to eating chocolate: from pleasure to aversion. *Brain* **124** (9) 1720–1733.

30   Smeets PA, de Graaf C, Stafleu A, van Osch MJ, Nievelstein RA & van der Grond J (2006) Effect of satiety on brain activation during chocolate tasting in men and women. *American Journal of Clinical Nutrition* **83** (6) 1297–1305.

31   Rogers PJ & Smit HJ (2000) Food craving and food 'addiction': a critical review of the evidence from a biopsychosocial perspective. *Pharmacology Biochemistry and Behavior* **66** (1) 3–14.

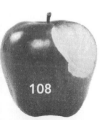

and the figure for women remained very similar at 90%.[32] There is, therefore, a suggestion that cultural differences affect the rates of men who confess to craving chocolate, whereas the women were consistent in both populations.

Countering the chocolate cravings/addiction

It is evident that there is no simple answer to whether or not chocolate is truly addictive or more of a craving. It is also evident that there will be no simple answer to preventing the craving/addiction. However, there are some steps that may help.

Gymnema sylvestre
Ingesting this herb can destroy the enjoyment value of chocolate, leaving the individual reluctant to eat more while the gymnema is active. However, gymnema's sweetness-blocking effects only last up to two hours so it is not a long-term solution; nor does it counter any perceived psychological dependence on chocolate.

Gymnema is reported to be able to decrease sugar absorption in the intestines and balance blood sugar. Due to this latter effect, it has been tested on patients with both insulin-dependent and non-insulin dependent diabetes, and has shown good results in reducing serum lipids and both fasting glucose and glycosylated haemoglobin (HbA1c) levels in Type II diabetic patients.[33,34]

However, it must be used with caution by anyone using glucose management drugs and with any other pre-existing health conditions, including pregnancy.

Interventions
Nutritional interventions
■ Reducing blood glucose imbalance in general may reduce cravings for high fat/high sugar foods. A nutritional approach to achieve this would therefore be beneficial in some cases.

32 Osman JL & Sobal J (2006) Chocolate cravings in American and Spanish individuals: biological and cultural influences. *Appetite* **47** (3) 290–301.

33 Shanmugasundaram ERB, Rajeswari G, Baskaran K, Rajesh Kumar BR & Radha Shanmugasundaram K (1990) Use of gymnema sylvestre leaf extract in the control of blood glucose in insulin-dependent diabetes mellitus. *Journal of Ethnopharmacology* **30** (3) 281–294.

34 Baskaran K, Kizar Ahamath B, Radha Shanmugasundara MK & Shanmugasundaram ERB (1990) Antidiabetic effect of a leaf extract from Gymnema sylvestre in non-insulin-dependent diabetes mellitus patients. *Journal of Ethnopharmacology* **30** (3) 295–305.

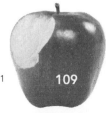

- If intestinal permeability is suspected then the casomorphins (from dairy) may also be involved in the 'addiction' and therefore healing the 'leaky gut' would be another beneficial intervention.

- Nutritional approaches to improving mood and hormone fluctuations may also achieve concomitant reduction in chocolate consumption.

- Balancing leptin levels: leptin helps to control appetite and is affected by steroid hormones in the body, so balancing leptin may happen as a side result of balancing hormone fluctuations.

None of these are independent of each other. In functional medicine terms, they would all be addressed together to achieve an overall balance in sugar metabolism, which may potentially reduce the perceived need for chocolate.

Psychotherapeutic interventions

As with other addictive behaviours, certain forms of re-directional therapy may have an application for chocolate 'addiction'. Types of cognitive behavioural therapy that include motivational enhancement, changing the response to the cue/stimulus and self-control training may all be of use. On the more complementary side, neuro-linguistic programming (NLP) may also be useful.

Self-help interventions

- **Only eat chocolate after a meal:** It has been shown that satiety has an effect on the craving and enjoyment of chocolate, so eating it after a meal is likely to reduce the amount consumed at any one sitting.

- **Exercise:** As well as eating, exercise is able to produce the natural endorphins that make us feel good. Therefore, this is a viable alternative to eating chocolate to produce the same endorphin 'high', and one that is a healthier alternative, which is likely to be accompanied by other health benefits as well.

- **Pharmaceutical drugs:** The use of naloxone has shown a reduction in cravings for addictive drugs. Since there are neurobiological elements of overlap with drug addiction and chocolate 'addiction', it is likely that blocking D2-dopamine receptors may also reduce cravings for chocolate and other high fat/high sugar foods. This may be a useful application in binge eaters and obese individuals who have particular issues with chocolate and other highly calorific foods associated with pleasure/reward.

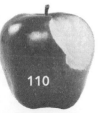

Box 5.2: NLP case study

Dorothy, 40, was concerned about her 'addiction' to chocolate. If there was any chocolate in the house she would be compelled to eat it and felt she was unable to moderate this need. In an NLP therapy session, her obsession with chocolate was traced back to her first blissful experience of it (a Heinz chocolate pudding form of baby food). The therapeutic intervention aimed to change her perception of chocolate to being 'just a food'. Dorothy now equates it with peas; in other words, it is now no more or less enjoyable than peas. She can still enjoy some chocolate but she no longer experiences insatiable cravings. This change has lasted for over a year.

Further reading

Some of this chapter is based on Chocolate Part II – Psychosomatic mood enhancer? by Ann Woodriff Beirne, which was first published in *The Nutrition Practitioner* **7** (2).

Chapter 6

Essential fatty acids and addictive disorders

Alexandra J Richardson

Introduction

The term 'addictive disorders' covers a wide range of conditions and extends well beyond substance use and dependence. Defining addiction is not easy but central to it are persistent patterns of dysfunctional and self-damaging behaviour, which are driven by powerful cravings, compulsions and/or impulses that the individual finds difficult or impossible to resist. Some eating disorders appear to involve addictive behaviour patterns and serious substance use or dependence is almost always accompanied by one or more of a wide range of other psychological disorders.

In this chapter the role of dietary fats in addictive disorders will be explored with specific reference to the potential importance of omega-3 and omega-6 polyunsaturates. These are the only fats that are 'dietary essentials' and they are critical in brain development and functioning. Many different psychological disorders have now been linked to deficiencies or imbalances involving omega-3 and/or omega-6 fats. Impulsivity and/or poor emotional self-regulation are associated with many of these conditions, just as they are with substance use disorders. The idea that fatty acid abnormalities may play some part in addictive disorders therefore seems well worth considering.

No nutrients operate in isolation so to place undue focus on any single nutrient (or group of nutrients) is not usually helpful. By definition, an adequate supply of all the essential micronutrients (eg. vitamins A, C and D) is required for physical and mental health, as well as a good balance of macronutrients ie. protein, carbohydrate, fat and dietary fibre. These are best provided through a varied and well-balanced diet that includes a wide range of fresh or relatively unprocessed foods, as illustrated by the Eatwell Plate (see Chapter 3). However, the Eatwell Plate is far from satisfactory with regard to guidance on the consumption of fats, as it groups fatty foods together with sugary foods as a category that should be limited, thus reinforcing the widely held misconception that 'all fat is bad'.

The truth is that there are many different types of dietary fats and they each have very different implications for our health. This is particularly true of mental health because 60% of the brain's dry mass is fat. The type and quality of fats in our diet, and their relative proportions, are therefore absolutely critical to brain development and functioning.

As a result of the industrialisation of our food supply, there have been huge changes in the fatty acid composition of diets in developed countries over the last 50–100 years. A consequence of this is that the dietary ratio of omega-6 to omega-3 polyunsaturates now far exceeds the ratios of between 1:1 and 4:1, which prevailed in the hunter-gatherer diets on which modern humans evolved. There is also good evidence that this relative lack of omega-3 (and the corresponding excess of omega-6) has contributed to the dramatic increases in the rates of many physical and mental health disorders in the developed world.[1]

Addictive disorders

■ Addiction is difficult to define but substance use and dependence are strongly associated with many other forms of psychological disorder, notably attention deficit hyperactivity disorder (ADHD), depression, anxiety, eating disorders, some personality disorders and most forms of psychosis.

■ These associations may reflect attempts at self-medication for these conditions and/or shared underlying risk factors (which may be genetic or environmental).

■ One environmental factor that raises the risk of having an addictive disorder or other psychological disorders is malnutrition in early life. This can have lifelong effects on gene expression, some of which can be passed on to future generations.

1   Simopoulos AP (2002) The importance of the ratio of omega-6/omega-3 essential fatty acids. *Biomedical Pharmacotherapy* **56** 365–379

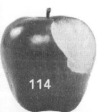

■ Improving the nutritional status of mothers before conception and during pregnancy would help to reduce the huge and increasing burden of mental health disorders, which has now overtaken that of physical health disorders in the UK and other developed countries.

The mechanisms underlying addiction are complex and while some addictive behaviours clearly involve known biochemical and physiological mechanisms (as indicated by increasing tolerance and/or physical withdrawal symptoms), others appear primarily to reflect the power of repeated associations and learned habits. Although, in practice, the value of such distinctions may be questionable, formal psychiatric classification systems – such as the widely used *Diagnostic and Statistical Manual of Mental Disorders* (DSM-IV-TR)[2] – now tend to use diagnoses such as 'substance use' and 'substance dependence' disorders for persistent patterns of problematic behaviour relating to the use of alcohol, tobacco, recreational drugs, solvents or other substances.

Separate diagnostic classifications are used for eating disorders but there is a good case for arguing that both 'binge eating' (as found in bulimia and many cases of obesity) and anorexia typically involve patterns of feelings, thoughts and behaviours with respect to food that meet most – if not all – criteria for addiction or substance dependence, as discussed in detail in Chapter 4. Addictive behaviour patterns can also be seen with respect to many other activities that do not involve food or other substances, with common examples including excessive gambling, spending, sex or internet use.

Substance use or dependence frequently co-occurs with eating disorders and other forms of addictive behaviour, thus raising the possibility that some people simply have 'addictive personalities'. However, no 'addictive personality' traits have been identified as such. Instead, a number of different traits – including impulsivity, sensation-seeking and anxiety – can increase the predisposition towards substance use disorders. These traits can be highly adaptive in some circumstances, but in others they can lead to difficulties with emotional self-regulation, which is usually a key element in substance use and dependence. There is a wide range of other psychological disorders in which these same traits feature; and unsurprisingly, substance use disorders are particularly common in people with these conditions. Attention deficit hyperactivity disorder (ADHD) increases the risk of all substance use disorders[3] but increased risks are also found in many other conditions, notably

2   American Psychiatric Association (2000) *Diagnostic and Statistical Manual of Mental Disorders (Revised 4th edition)*. Washington DC: APA.

3   Wilens TE, Martelon M, Joshi G, Bateman C, Fried R, Petty C & Biederman J (2011) Does ADHD predict substance use disorders? A 10-year follow-up study of young adults with ADHD. *Journal of the American Academy of Child & Adolescent Psychiatry* **50** (6) 543–553.

depression and other mood disorders, post-traumatic stress disorder, anxiety disorders, some types of personality disorder and psychosis.[4]

The strong overlaps between substance use disorders and psychological disorders may of course reflect attempts at 'self-medication', but they could also reflect common underlying risk factors. Genetic factors clearly have a role, but the genetic risks for most psychological disorders are multifactorial and involve many different (normal) genes, each contributing only small effects and interacting with a wide range of environmental factors. Low socioeconomic status and early emotional deprivation are known to increase the risk of all of these conditions. Children born to mothers who abuse alcohol or other substances are particularly vulnerable to developing substance use disorders themselves – reflecting both genetic factors and the many adverse environmental influences that these children experience from the outset.

One important adverse environmental influence of low socioeconomic status is a relatively poor diet, which increases the risk of essential micronutrient deficiencies. This can be particularly damaging in early life as prenatal malnutrition will compound the toxic effects of alcohol and other substances on early brain development. In recent years it has been shown that maternal nutritional status at conception and during pregnancy can permanently modify the expression of many genes in offspring – an effect known as 'nutritional programming'.[5] Mothers' diets before and during pregnancy therefore have long-term effects on their children's health and well-being and furthermore, some environmentally-induced changes in gene expression (known as 'epigenetic' effects) are also heritable.

Studies of children conceived or born during the Dutch famine of 1944–45 (ie. children subjected to serious prenatal malnutrition in terms of energy and protein as well as micronutrients) found that, as adults, these individuals showed higher rates of addictive disorders (as well as many other forms of psychological disorder) when compared with matched controls.[6] While these children obviously represent extreme cases, they provide proof of concept that early nutrition is an important determinant of future mental health. This means that efforts to reduce the overall

---

4   Chen KW, Banducci AN, Guller L, Macatee RJ, Lavelle A, Daughters SB & Lejuez CW (2011) An examination of psychiatric co-morbidities as a function of gender and substance type within an inpatient substance use treatment program. *Drug and Alcohol Dependence* April 21 [Epub ahead of print]

5   Langley-Evans SC & McMullen S (2010) Developmental origins of adult disease. *Medical Principles and Practice* **19** (2) 87–98.

6   Franzek EJ, Sprangers N, Janssens AC, Van Duijn CM & Van De Wetering BJ (2008) Prenatal exposure to the 1944-45 Dutch 'hunger winter' and addiction later in life. *Addiction* **103** (3) 433–438.

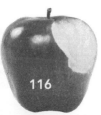

prevalence and severity of substance use disorders, and the mental health problems with which they are associated, are likely to have limited success unless they include a focus on prevention, in terms of improving the nutrition of mothers before and during pregnancy. This would not only help to support optimal brain development in their children but would also be expected to improve the mother's own mental health and functioning, which is itself a major influence on children's development and well-being.

The scale of mental health problems facing the UK and other developed countries is immense, and the burden of these has now overtaken that of physical health disorders. According to government figures, the cost of mental health disorders in the UK in 2007 totalled £77 billion (more than the cost of heart disease and cancer combined) and by 2010 this had risen to £105 billion. Back in the 1970s, professor Michael Crawford – one of the early pioneers of research into omega-3 and omega-6 fats – warned that unless action was taken to improve the quality and balance of the fats provided by modern western diets, brain disorders would overtake cardiovascular disease in terms of their health burden.[7] We now appear to have passed that point.

Essential fatty acids

■ The only essential fats are omega-3 and omega-6 polyunsaturates but in each case it is the longer chain, highly unsaturated fatty acids (HUFA) that are biologically important, not the shorter chain omega-3 or omega-6 fats.

■ Conversion of short-chain omega-3 and omega-6 fats into the respective HUFA is inefficient and unreliable so adequate dietary sources of pre-formed HUFA are preferable. Meat, eggs and dairy products provide pre-formed omega-6 HUFA, but only fish and seafood provide the key omega-3 HUFA.

■ Modern western diets provide an excess of omega-6 over omega-3 – both the shorter chain forms (found in vegetable oils) and the pre-formed HUFA. This increases risks for a wide range of physical and mental health disorders.

---

7   See 'World's foremost omega-3 experts predict mental health epidemic' – report on the 'Celebration of DHA' Press conference, 26 May 2010, Royal Society of Medicine. Available at: www.fabresearch.org/1462

- Adequate supplies of omega-3 and omega-6 HUFA, and an appropriate balance between these, are essential for normal brain development and function. These fats directly influence brain structure and substances made from them are key regulators of many chemical signalling systems in the brain, as well as influencing blood flow, hormone balance and immune system function.

Only two types of fat are 'dietary essentials' – meaning that, like vitamins, they are absolutely critical for our health, but we cannot make them so they must be provided by the food we eat. These essential fats are the omega-3 and omega-6 polyunsaturated fatty acids (PUFA) but there are many different forms of each, as seen in Table 6.1.

Table 6.1: Omega-6 and omega-3 polyunsaturated fatty acids

Omega-6 series		Enzymes involved in HUFA synthesis	Omega-3 series	
Linoleic (LA)	18:2		Alpha-linolenic (ALA)	18:3
↓		Delta 6-desaturase	↓	
Gamma-linolenic (GLA)	18:3		Octadecatetraenoic	18:4
↓		Elongase	↓	
Dihomogamma-linolenic (DGLA)	20:3		Eicosatetraenoic	20:4
↓		Delta 5-desaturase	↓	
Arachidonic (AA)	20:4		Eicosapentaenoic (EPA)	20:5
↓		Elongase	↓	
Adrenic	22:4		Docosapentaenoic (DPA)	22:5
↓		Elongase, Delta 6-desaturase, Beta-oxidation	↓	
Docosapentaenoic (DPA)	22:5		Docosahexaenoic (DHA)	22:6

The simplest, shorter-chain forms of omega-6 and omega-3 polyunsaturates are linoleic acid (LA) and alpha-linolenic acid (ALA). However, it is the more highly unsaturated fatty acids (HUFA) that are most important for brain development and function – notably dihomogamma-linolenic

(DGLA) and arachidonic (AA) (omega-6) and eicosapentaenoic (EPA) and docosahexaenoic (DHA) (omega-3). These HUFA can in theory be synthesised from the shorter chain forms via processes of de-saturation (insertion of a double-bond between the carbon atoms in the chain) and elongation (adding two carbon atoms to the fatty acid chain). However, the conversion of LA and ALA to the respective HUFA is relatively slow and inefficient in humans, so pre-formed HUFA from dietary sources is preferable to ensure an adequate supply of these vital nutrients.

- AA and DHA are major structural components of neuronal membranes (making up 15–20% of the dry mass of the brain and more than 30% of the retina).

- EPA and DGLA are also crucial but play functional rather than structural roles.

- EPA, DGLA and AA are needed to manufacture eicosanoids – hormone-like substances including prostaglandins, leukotrienes, and thromboxanes. These and other HUFA derivatives (including some from DHA) play critical roles in the moment-by-moment regulation of a very wide range of brain and body functions.

Both omega-3 and omega-6 are needed in our diets as they are not interconvertible within the body. The balance between omega-3 and omega-6 is also crucial as this affects the functioning of almost all brain and body systems.

Dietary sources of omega-3 and omega-6 fats

Omega-6

The simplest (shortest chain) omega-6 fat is linoleic acid (LA), which is found in all vegetable oils, nuts, seeds and grains. It can be found in most processed foods (see Box 6.1). As a result, modern western-type diets usually contain excessive amounts of LA. In an average US diet, LA contributes almost 10% of all energy (calories), compared with a recommended intake of around 2%.

> ### Box 6.1: Linoleic acid: an omega-6 consumed to excess
>
> The simplest omega-6 fat, linoleic acid (LA), is found in:
>
> - all vegetable oils (such as corn, sunflower, safflower and soy bean oil etc) as well as all grains, seeds and nuts.
>
> LA is therefore abundant in most processed and commercially produced foods, such as:
>
> - margarines (and other non-dairy substitutes for milk, cream, yogurt, butter or cheese)
> - salad dressings and sauces
> - biscuits, confectionery, cakes, pastries, crisps and other snacks or desserts
> - fried foods, takeaways and ready meals.

The longer chain omega-6 HUFA, arachidonic acid (AA), is the most biologically important of the omega-6 fats. It is found pre-formed in meat, eggs and dairy produce so in developed countries it is usually abundant in all but the strictest vegan diets.

Omega-3

The simplest of the omega-3 fats, alpha-linolenic acid (ALA), is found in green leafy vegetables and some nut and seed oils. Flax (linseed) oil is a particularly rich source of ALA, but small quantities are provided by rapeseed oil, walnuts and pumpkin seeds. Importantly, almost all vegetable oils provide much more omega-6 (LA) than omega-3 (ALA), with flax oil being the notable exception.

The biologically important omega-3 are the longer-chain HUFA, specifically EPA and DHA. Fish and seafood are the only natural foods that provide these fatty acids pre-formed in any appreciable quantities. Traces of EPA are found in meat from grass-fed animals and some DHA can be obtained from organ meats, or eggs from birds that eat seeds like flax or herbs such as purslane, which are rich in ALA. EPA and DHA can also be derived from some forms of algae and can be found in particular supplements and fortified food.

Omega-3 and omega-6: the long and the short of it

As emphasised above, it is the longer chain, more highly unsaturated fatty acids (HUFA) of each series that are the most important for human health ie. these are the ones that are truly 'essential' in terms of their biological functions. The shorter chain omega-3 and omega-6 (ALA and LA respectively) do not have the same health benefits. In fact, their main value to humans appears to be as raw materials for making the longer chain fats of the same series. In practice, however, the process of synthesising the longer chain omega-3 and omega-6 HUFA within the body is very unreliable in humans, so a direct dietary supply of these essential fats in a 'pre-formed' state is preferable.

The efficiency of this conversion pathway differs between individuals and factors that can affect this include:

- **genetics:** genetic variation in the rate-limiting enzymes (known as fatty acid desaturases or FADS) means that conversion efficiency varies with ancestry

- **sex:** on average, females are better at this conversion for hormonal reasons, so males are more vulnerable to HUFA deficiencies, other things being equal[8]

- **age:** conversion is thought to be less efficient in young children and older adults

- **dietary fat intake:** the relative intakes of shorter-chain omega-6 (LA) and omega-3 (ALA) affect conversion of each, as they compete for the enzymes involved

- **availability of essential co-factors:** many different vitamins and minerals are needed as 'co-factors' for the FADS enzymes – including vitamins A, B3, B6 and C, as well as zinc and magnesium

- **other lifestyle factors:** stress, and some viral infections, can impair conversion.

Synthesis of the omega-3 HUFA from ALA appears to be particularly poor, probably reflecting competition for enzymes against the excess of LA in modern, western-type diets. Humans can make some EPA from ALA,

---

8   Giltay EJ, Gooren LJ, Toorians AW, Katan MB & Zock PL (2004) Docosahexaenoic acid concentrations are higher in women than in men because of estrogenic effects. American *Journal of Clinical Nutrition* **80** 1167–1174.

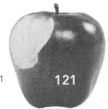

but this conversion is inefficient (around 5%) and the synthesis of DHA from ALA is virtually negligible (<1%). This has important implications for vegetarians and those who do not eat fish and seafood – the main dietary sources of EPA and DHA. With respect to omega-3 fats, therefore, the international scientific consensus is that pre-formed DHA is in fact a dietary essential for humans.[9]

Essential fats and the brain

Omega-3 and omega-6 HUFA should make up 15–20% of the brain's dry mass because they are key components of all brain and nerve cell membranes. Two HUFA are particularly important for normal brain structure: the omega-6 AA, and the omega-3 DHA. These increase the fluidity of cell membranes, which is essential for normal cell signalling. DHA alone should make up 30–50% of the retina and this omega-3 HUFA is absolutely critical for normal development and functioning of the visual system.[10]

For normal brain function, omega-3 and omega-6 fatty acids (and the balance between them) are important for many different reasons.

- Three of these fatty acids (the omega-3 EPA, and the omega-6 AA and DGLA) act as raw materials for a huge array of regulatory substances (known as 'eicosanoids') that influence hormonal, cardiovascular and immune system functioning. Crucially:
  - the omega-6 AA gives rise to eicosanoids that are pro-thrombotic (ie. they promote blood clotting) and pro-inflammatory
  - by contrast, the omega-3 EPA gives rise to eicosanoids that are anti-coagulant (ie. they reduce blood clotting) and act to reduce inflammation.
- Other substances made from the long-chain omega-3 EPA and DHA also have anti-inflammatory actions and some help to protect brain cells in other ways (examples include 'resolvins' made from EPA and 'neuroprotectins' from DHA).[11]

9   Brenna JT, Salem N Jr, Sinclair AJ & Cunnane SC (2009) Alpha-linolenic acid supplementation and conversion to n-3 long-chain polyunsaturated fatty acids in humans. *Prostaglandins, Leukotrienes and Essential Fatty Acids (PLEFA)* 80 (2–3) 85–91.

10   Uauy R, Hoffman DR, Peirano P, Birch DG & Birch EE (2001) Essential fatty acids in visual and brain development. *Lipids* **36** (9) 885–895.

11   Serhan CN (2005) Novel eicosanoid and docosanoid mediators: resolvins, docosatrienes, and neuroprotectins. *Current Opinion in Clinical Nutrition and Metabolic Care* **8** (2) 115–121.

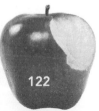

- EPA, DHA and AA regulate the transcription and expression of numerous genes in the body and brain.

- AA, EPA and DHA and their many derivatives also influence the levels and activity of many neurotransmitters (ie. the substances used in brain cell signalling), such as dopamine (involved in arousal, motivation and 'reward' signalling) and serotonin (implicated in mood and numerous other brain and body functions).

- AA is the source of the endogenous cannabinoids (or 'endocannabinoids') – substances produced within the body that activate the same receptors as the active ingredients in cannabis (marijuana). Endocannabinoid concentrations influence many different aspects of psychological functioning, including sensitivity to pain, perceptual and attentional processing, motor control, memory and other aspects of cognitive functioning.

Omega-3/omega-6 balance

Because omega-3 and omega-6 fats play so many different roles in the body and brain, the ratio of these fats in the diet affects almost every aspect of physical and mental health.

As emphasised above, substances made from the omega-3 HUFA EPA have anti-inflammatory and anti-thrombotic effects, while those made from the main omega-6 HUFA AA (via exactly the same enzymes) are pro-inflammatory and pro-thrombotic. This simple fact helps to explain why the elevated omega-6/omega-3 ratio in modern, western-type diets (and specifically, a high AA/EPA ratio) helps to promote inflammatory disorders and cardiovascular disease (to which low-grade, chronic inflammation contributes).

Modern western diets are particularly rich in the shorter-chain omega-6 LA and very low in the corresponding omega-3 ALA. Under these circumstances, 'good conversion' of short to long chain polyunsaturates can actually be a disadvantage. For example, it has recently been shown that African Americans are more likely to be 'good converters' than those of European descent.[12] As a result, African Americans show significantly

---

12   Mathias RA, Sergeant S, Ruczinski I, Torgerson DG, Hugenschmidt CE, Kubala M, Vaidya D, Suktitipat B, Ziegler JT, Ivester P, Case D, Yanek LR, Freedman BI, Rudock ME, Barnes KC, Langefeld CD, Becker LC, Bowden DW, Becker DM & Chilton FH (2011) The impact of FADS genetic variants on n-6 polyunsaturated fatty acid metabolism in African Americans. *BMC Genetics* **12** (1) 50.

higher blood AA concentrations than European Americans and this probably helps to explain why they are at a particularly high risk for heart disease, inflammatory disorders and many other so-called 'western diseases'.

Inflammation has effects on the brain and nervous system because they share many chemical signalling systems. The pro-inflammatory bias induced by diets rich in omega-6 fats is thought to be one contributory factor to depression for this reason.[13] The dietary omega-3/omega-6 balance also affects the functioning of most 'classical' neurotransmitters (such as dopamine, serotonin, noradrenaline and NMDA). It is also fundamental to the more recently discovered endocannabinoid system, adding yet another reason why dietary fat intake is such an important modulator of brain function.

The relevance of essential fatty acids to addictive disorders

- Adequate supplies – and an appropriate balance – of HUFA in early life is critical for normal brain development and functioning in later life. Prenatal HUFA deficiencies or imbalances and/or substitution of these with 'trans fats' have the potential to 'prime' the next generation for addictive and mental health disorders.

- Substance use has adverse effects on fatty acid and micronutrient status, directly affecting neurotransmitter systems and brain function.

- There is mounting evidence for fatty acid abnormalities in eating disorders and various other psychological disorders with which substance use is associated, including ADHD, depression, PTSD and schizophrenia.

Early life nutrition

Many studies now show that maternal dietary fat intake during pregnancy can have long-term consequences for brain structure and function. Most studies involve animals, but the findings indicate that consuming a modern, western-type diet high in processed foods (ie. rich in saturated fats and omega-6 from vegetable oils, with little or no omega-3) affects the brain development of the offspring in numerous ways that are likely to increase

13   Pascoe MC, Crewther SG, Carey LM & Crewther DP (2011) What you eat is what you are: a role for polyunsaturated fatty acids in neuroinflammation induced depression. *Clinical Nutrition* **30** (4) 407–415.

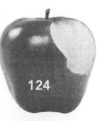

the vulnerability to substance use and other addictive disorders in later life. This kind of dietary fat intake in early life has been shown to increase anxiety and dysfunctional responses to stress (ie. poor emotional self-regulation)[14,15] and prenatal omega-3 deficiency is associated with increases in both depression and aggression in later life.[16]

Hydrogenated vegetable oils are particularly pernicious because they contain twisted, toxic versions of the natural omega-6 and omega-3 polyunsaturates, known as 'trans fats'. Despite the numerous serious health risks associated with consuming trans fats, they have not yet been banned in the UK and many other countries.[17] They are still found in margarines, spreads, snacks, biscuits, cakes, pastries and other highly processed foods including ready meals and takeaways (especially the cheaper varieties of all of these foods). The diets of most people with substance use disorders are likely to contain higher than average levels of trans fats.

Trans fats have long been known to raise the risk of diabetes, heart disease, stroke and cancer, among other serious physical health problems. New evidence has clearly shown that consuming trans fats also has detrimental effects on the brain. Repeated amphetamine exposure promotes hyperactivity and manic behaviour and a diet rich in trans fats amplifies this, whereas a diet low in omega-6 and rich in omega-3 fats (ie. the opposite of the typical 'junk food diet') is protective.[18]

Another important recent study has not only confirmed previous findings that omega-3 deficiency in early life causes depressive-like symptoms in animals, but has also shown that it permanently impairs endocannabinoid signalling in brain networks important for emotional regulation.[19]

14   Sullivan EL, Grayson B, Takahashi D, Robertson N, Maier A, Bethea CL, Smith MS, Coleman K & Grove KL (2010) Chronic consumption of a high fat diet during pregnancy causes perturbations in the serotonergic system and increased anxiety-like behaviour in non-human primate offspring. *Journal of Neuroscience* **3** (10) 3826–3830.

15   D'Asti E, Long H, Tremblay-Mercier J, Grajzer M, Cunnane SC, Di Marzo V & Walker CD (2010) Maternal dietary fat determines metabolic profile and the magnitude of endocannabinoid inhibition of the stress response in neonatal rat offspring. *Endocrinology* **151** (4) 1685–1694.

16   DeMar JC Jr, Ma K, Bell JM, Igarashi M, Greenstein D & Rapoport SI (2006) One generation of n-3 polyunsaturated fatty acid deprivation increases depression and aggression test scores in rats. *Journal of Lipid Research* **47** (1) 172–180.

17   Mozaffarian D & Stampfer MJ (2010) Removing industrial trans fat from foods. *BMJ* **340** 1826.

18   Trevizol F, Benvegnú DM, Barcelos RC, Boufleur N, Dolci GS, Müller LG, Pase CS, Reckziegel P, Dias VT, Segat H, Teixeira AM, Emanuelli T, Rocha JB & Bürger ME (2011) Comparative study between n-6, trans and n-3 fatty acids on repeated amphetamine exposure: a possible factor for the development of mania. *Pharmacology Biochemistry and Behavior* **97** (3) 560–565.

19   Lafourcade M, Larrieu T, Mato S, Duffaud A, Sepers M, Matias I, De Smedt-Peyrusse V, Labrousse VF, Bretillon L, Matute C, Rodríguez-Puertas R, Layé S & Manzoni OJ (2011) Nutritional omega-3 deficiency abolishes endocannabinoid-mediated neuronal functions. *Nature Neuroscience* **14** (3) 345–350.

It is well known that early emotional deprivation is a major risk factor for substance use and other addictive disorders. Less well known is that maternal dietary fat intake during pregnancy actually interacts with the effects of stress and emotional deprivation on mood and behaviour, leading to dysfunctional patterns of emotional responsivity that persist into adulthood. In a recent study it was shown that either early omega-3 deficiency or maternal deprivation led to increases in impulsivity and the response to reward, as assessed by sucrose consumption.[20] However, the combination of the two had a synergistic (multiplier) effect, increasing sucrose intake by 80% compared with control conditions. Furthermore, the effects of omega-3 deficiency on brain fatty acid composition (specifically the resulting increase in brain concentrations of the omega-6 AA) were also significantly amplified by the emotional stress of maternal deprivation. Thus omega-3 deficiency and known psychosocial stressors both have negative effects on brain development, but the combination of the two multiplies these. Behaviourally, the result is a dramatically increased vulnerability to traits such as impulsivity and reward sensitivity, which are known to contribute to 'addictive' behaviour patterns later in life.

Prenatal nutrition clearly has powerful effects but diet and lifestyle factors continue to impact on mental health throughout life. Of course, substance use and other forms of addiction often tend to lead to vicious downward spirals in this respect, but a key issue is the extent to which nutritional factors contribute to this, because diet is potentially easier to change than many of the other 'lifestyle' factors involved in addictive disorders.

Essential fatty acids and substance use disorders

Drinking and smoking deplete essential fatty acid store

Use of the legal drugs, alcohol and/or tobacco, is exceptionally common in people with other forms of addictive behaviours. Excessive alcohol intake reliably leads to deficiencies of both omega-3 and omega-6 HUFA. In developed

---

20 Mathieu G, Denis S, Lavialle M & Vancassel S (2008) Synergistic effects of stress and omega-3 fatty acid deprivation on emotional response and brain lipid composition in adult rats. *Prostaglandins, Leukotrienes and Essential Fatty Acids (PLEFA)* **78** (6) 391–401.

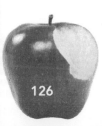

countries like the UK, heavy drinking is likely to reduce brain omega-3 concentrations in particular, simply because these are far less abundant in the diet than omega-6. Of course, excessive use of alcohol also depletes the body and brain of many other essential nutrients, so that anyone with chronic alcohol dependence is likely to become seriously malnourished over time.[21] In extreme cases this can lead to irreversible brain damage, as seen in Korsakoff's syndrome (involving profound memory impairments and motor co-ordination problems), caused by prolonged deficiency of thiamine (vitamin B1).

Smoking also depletes omega-3 and omega-6 HUFA stores as the many toxic substances in tobacco smoke increase oxidative stress, to which these fatty acids are particularly vulnerable.

Nutrients, drugs and neurotransmitters

Numerous illegal substances are used as recreational drugs and most impact on many different neurotransmitter systems. Common examples include:

■ amphetamines (speed), cocaine and similar substances, which stimulate *dopamine* receptors in particular

■ heroin, morphine, codeine and others, which primarily activate *opiate* receptors

■ MDMA (ecstasy), which activates some 5-HT (*serotonin*) receptors

■ cannabis or marijuana, which acts on receptors for the *endocannabinoids* (anandamide and 2-arachidonylglycerol (2-AG)).

All neurotransmitters have to be manufactured within the body or brain on an ongoing basis and both their production and their recycling depend critically on nutrition. Diet is the ultimate source of both the raw materials and the many co-factors needed to make, utilise, break down and recycle all neurotransmitters; hence any deficiencies or imbalances in essential nutrients can affect their availability.

The poor diet consumed by most substance users increases their risks of deficiencies in many essential micronutrients. Individual metabolic differences (owing to genetic, epigenetic or transient environmental influences) can also lead to some people having vastly differing nutrient requirements in order to maintain the same levels of neurotransmitter synthesis, release and re-uptake.

---

21   Lieber CS (1988) The influence of alcohol on nutritional status. *Nutrition Reviews* **46** (7) 241–254.

Omega-3 and omega-6 HUFA concentrations impact on almost all neurotransmitter systems, either directly or indirectly, so the availability of these fats in the diet – and the balance between them – has direct relevance for substance abuse of any kind, as well as for psychological disorders in which these signalling systems are implicated.

■ Chronic omega-3 deficiencies in early life reduce dopamine and its binding to D2 receptors both in frontal cortex and other brain regions, and are associated with the kinds of attentional and behavioural dysfunctions seen in ADHD.[22] Subsequent dietary supplementation appears to remedy some of the dopaminergic abnormalities induced by omega-3 deficiencies during early development, but not others.[23]

■ Dietary fat intake – and in particular the omega-3/omega-6 balance – is a major determinant of endocannabinoid concentrations, because the two main endocannabinoids (anandamide and 2-arachidonyl glycerol or 2-AG) are both derived from the omega-6 HUFA AA.[24] As we shall see, the cannabinoids have important implications not only for substance use, but for many other psychological disorders including eating disorders, mood disorders and psychosis.

Dietary intervention studies of people with substance use disorders are few as they are an extremely difficult group to study given their often chaotic lifestyles. Only one small randomised controlled trial of omega-3 supplementation in this population has been published to date involving 24 patients undergoing rehabilitation for substance abuse. Over the three-month treatment period, patients who received 3g a day of long-chain omega-3 from fish oils (EPA and DHA) reported progressive reductions in their feelings of anxiety compared with the patients who received placebo treatment.[25] This group difference in anxiety was significant, and although dietary supplementation was discontinued at the three-month point, the reductions in anxiety following omega-3 treatment were maintained, such that the group difference was still significant three months later.

Self-reported feelings of anger were also monitored in this study and these too were significantly lower following omega-3 treatment than placebo

22   Zimmer L, Vancassel S, Cantagrel S, Breton P, Delamanche S, Guilloteau D, Durand G & Chalon S (2002) The dopamine mesocorticolimbic pathway is affected by deficiency in n-3 polyunsaturated fatty acids. *American Journal of Clinical Nutrition* **75** 662–667.

23   Levant B, Radel JD & Carlson SE (2004) Decreased brain docosahexaenoic acid during development alters dopamine-related behaviors in adult rats that are differentially affected by dietary remediation. *Behavioural Brain Research* **152** 49–57.

24   Banni S & Di Marzo V (2010) Effect of dietary fat on endocannabinoids and related mediators: consequences on energy homeostasis, inflammation and mood. *Molecular Nutrition & Food Research* **54** (1) 82–92.

25   Buydens-Branchey L & Branchey M (2006) n-3 polyunsaturated fatty acids decrease anxiety feelings in a population of substance abusers. *Journal of Clinical Psychopharmacology* **26** (6) 661–665.

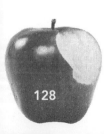

at the end of the three-month treatment period. Again, this reduction
in feelings of anger was sustained for a further three months after the
supplementation was stopped. It was also noted that, before treatment
began, patients with a history of assaultive behaviour had significantly
lower fish and omega-3 PUFA intakes than those without such a history.[26]

Essential fatty acids in other 'addictive disorders'

Relative omega-3 deficiencies have now been implicated in almost all of
the psychological disorders in which addictive behaviour patterns are
particularly common, including some eating disorders, ADHD and related
neurodevelopmental disorders, antisocial and other personality disorders,
depression and other mood disorders, and the schizophrenia spectrum.[27,28]

Obesity and compulsive overeating

As discussed in Chapter 4, some forms of eating disorder have many
apparent parallels with substance use and dependence.[29] This is not really
surprising as many of the biological factors that affect appetite and satiety
(and thus food intake) are intrinsically linked with various chemical
'reward' systems that operate both in the brain and elsewhere in the body.
These same chemical reward systems appear to be involved in almost all
addictive behaviours. Furthermore, the same brain regions associated with
addictive drug cravings and the motivational drive to use these are also
activated in humans experiencing emotional eating episodes and/or loss of
control with respect to food intake.[30]

Food cravings almost always involve highly palatable processed and refined
foods that are high in fat, sugar and/or salt. Good evidence now indicates that

26 Buydens-Branchey L & Branchey M (2008) Long-chain n-3 polyunsaturated fatty acids decrease feelings
of anger in substance abusers. *Psychiatry Research* **157** (1–3) 95–104.

27 Vaddadi K (2006) Essential fatty acids and mental illness. *International Review of Psychiatry* **18** (2)
81–186.

28 Associate Parliamentary Food and Health Forum (2008) The Links between Diet and Behaviour: The
influence of nutrition on mental health. Available at: http://www.fabresearch.org/1178 (accessed August 9 2011).

29 Taylor VH, Curtis CM & Davis C (2010) The obesity epidemic: the role of addiction. *Canadian Medical
Association Journal (CMAJ)* **182** (4) 327–328.

30 Wang GJ, Yang J, Volkow ND, Telang F, Ma Y, Zhu W, Wong CT, Tomasi D, Thanos PK & Fowler JS (2006)
Gastric stimulation in obese subjects activates the hippocampus and other regions involved in brain reward
circuitry. *Proceedings of the National Academy of Sciences USA* **103** (42) 15641–15645.

the consumption of a modern western-type diet that is rich in these kinds of foods can seriously distort the usual self-regulating feedback mechanisms that influence appetite and satiety (involving hormones such as insulin, leptin and ghrelin),[31] and also has detrimental effects on energy metabolism and motivation to exercise. The result is 'obligate weight gain' for essentially metabolic reasons (ie. 'laziness' and 'greed' are secondary consequences of this kind of diet) leading to obesity and/or other forms of eating disorders.

There is evidence that sugar may have 'addictive' properties[32,33] but it is possible that the fat content of foods high in fat, sugar and/or salt may also contribute to food cravings and overeating. 'High fat' in this context usually means high in short chain omega-6 from vegetable oils, with little or no omega-3, although the saturated fat content may also be high in some cases – for example, from butter, cream or cheese.

Deficiencies in omega-3 relative to omega-6 HUFA can affect appetite and food intake via their effects on cannabinoid signalling.[34] The endocannabinoids are orexigenic (acting to increase appetite) and they appear to increase the preference for sweet tastes. Furthermore, both of these effects oppose those of leptin (a hormone important in limiting food intake) with which endocannabinoid levels are inversely correlated.[35] An excessive dietary intake of omega-6 fats, as found in modern western-type diets, increases circulating levels of 2-AG and anandamide, and this has now been shown to increase tendencies towards overeating – particularly of highly palatable foods – and to promote obesity.

Anorexia

Most individuals with anorexia are fat-phobic, so severe omega-3 PUFA deficiency is highly likely to develop during self-induced starvation, especially if the little food they do consume is typical of a modern, western-type diet (rich in omega-6 PUFAs, saturates and trans-fats).

31   Lustig RH (2006) Childhood obesity: behavioral aberration or biochemical drive? Reinterpreting the first law of thermodynamics. *Nature Clinical Practice Endocrinology & Metabolism* 2 447–458.

32   Colantuoni C, Rada P, McCarthy J, Patten C, Avena NM, Chadeayne A & Hoebel BG (2002). Evidence that intermittent, excessive sugar intake causes endogenous opioid dependence. *Obesity Research* 10 (6) 478–488.

33   Spangler R, Wittkowski KM, Goddard NL, Avena NM, Hoebel BG & Leibowitz SF (2004) Opiate-like effects of sugar on gene expression in reward areas of the rat brain. *Brain Research and Molelcular Brain Research* 124 (2) 134–142.

34   Kirkham TC & Tucci SA (2006) Endocannabinoids in appetite control and the treatment of obesity. *CNS & Neurological Disorders – Drug Targets* 5 (3) 272–292.

35   Yoshida R, Ohkuri T, Jyotaki M, Yasuo T, Horio N, Yasumatsu K, Sanematsu K, Shigemura N, Yamamoto T, Margolskee RF & Ninomiya Y (2010) Endocannabinoids selectively enhance sweet taste. *Proceedings of the National Academy of Sciences USA* 107 (2) 935–939.

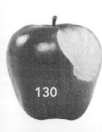

Standard re-feeding programmes do not currently consider omega-3 PUFA intake, which may lead to further omega-3 deficiency during weight restoration. Deficiencies of EPA and DHA are associated with a wide range of perceptual, cognitive, behavioural and emotional disturbances, which could plausibly help to maintain the dysfunctional beliefs and behaviours that characterise anorexia. As yet, however, there are only two published treatment studies of anorexia involving omega-3 supplementation.

- In a small open-label pilot study, seven young patients with anorexia nervosa received 1g a day of the long chain omega-3 EPA in addition to standard treatment; they were followed up for three months, by which time three had recovered and four had improved.[36]

- A single case reported that supplementation with EPA and multivitamins led to rapid clinical improvement.[37]

Given the seriousness of anorexia and the relatively high failure rate seen in conventional treatment, this pilot data is encouraging. Although they are obviously very preliminary and do not provide evidence of efficacy, omega-3 are safe and have many health benefits (and serious deficiencies carry many risks to physical health, which are already elevated in anorexic individuals). Randomised controlled trials of omega-3 LC-PUFA as an adjunct to standard treatments are clearly needed but in the meanwhile, their clinical use can easily be justified on physical health grounds.

Anorexia is of course likely to lead to deficiencies or insufficiencies of almost all essential nutrients. Zinc is particularly important in anorexia because deficiencies can further impair appetite and reduce food intake. In controlled trials zinc supplementation has been shown to improve the rate of recovery of anorexic patients, not only by increasing their weight gain but also by reducing their levels of anxiety and depression.[38]

ADHD

Abnormally low blood concentrations of omega-3 HUFA (and often – but not always – a corresponding excess of omega-6 HUFA) have repeatedly been reported in association with ADHD and related conditions.[39] The evidence

36 Ayton AK, Azaz A & Horrobin DF (2004) A pilot open case series of Ethyl-EPA supplementation in the treatment of anorexia nervosa. *Prostaglandins, Leukotrienes and Essential Fatty Acids (PLEFA)* **71** (4) 205–209.

37 Ayton AK, Azaz A & Horrobin DF (2004) Rapid improvement of severe anorexia nervosa during treatment with ethyl-eicosapentaenoate and micronutrients. *European Psychiatry* **19** (5) 317–319.

38 Su JC & Birmingham CL (2002) Zinc supplementation in the treatment of anorexia nervosa. *Eating and Weight Disorders* **7** (1) 20–22.

39 Richardson AJ (2006) Omega-3 fatty acids in ADHD and related neurodevelopmental disorders. *International Review of Psychiatry* **18** (2) 155–172.

from controlled treatment trials to date is more mixed, but these remain few and small with different populations, treatment formulations and dosages, and outcome measures. Dietary supplementation with omega-3 HUFA (EPA and DHA) appears to benefit at least a subset of those with ADHD-type symptoms, and two sets of characteristics appear to predict a good response:

1. poor emotional self-regulation eg. anxiety and/or mood disorders, including depression, bipolar disorder and 'oppositional defiant disorder'

2. specific learning difficulties, particularly dyslexia or dyspraxia.

The first of these has obvious relevance to substance use disorders and ADHD is such a heterogeneous condition that further research would do well to focus on specific subgroups such as this.

Depression and other mood disorders

Substantial evidence – both direct and indirect – indicates that low dietary intakes of the long-chain omega-3 fats found in fish and seafood (EPA and DHA) contribute to depression and other mood disorders.[40] Many randomised controlled trials (RCT) have now shown that adjunctive treatment with omega-3 HUFA (EPA and DHA) can be of therapeutic benefit in depression. By 2006 this evidence was already sufficient that the American Psychiatric Association made a treatment recommendation that all patients with either major depression or psychotic disorders should consume at least 1,000mg per day of EPA and DHA (equivalent to three or more servings of oily fish per week) in addition to standard treatment.[41]

Many more treatment trials have been carried out since then and subsequent meta-analyses have confirmed that an increased intake of long-chain omega-3 (and particularly EPA rather than DHA) is effective in reducing symptoms in major depression,[42] although this has not yet been recognised (or even acknowledged) in the latest NICE guidelines.

For bipolar disorder, a Cochrane review found too few studies for meta-analysis, although several early trials suggested benefits and the one high-quality trial showed that either 1g per day or 2g per day of pure EPA was

40   Hibbeln J (2009) Depression, suicide and deficiencies of omega-3 essential fatty acids in modern diets. *World Review of Nutrition and Dietetics* **99** 17–30.

41   Freeman MP, Hibbeln JR, Wisner KL, Davis JM, Mischoulon D, Peet M, Keck PE, Marangel LB, Richardson AJ, Lake J & Stoll AL (2006) Omega-3 fatty acids: evidence basis for treatment and future research in psychiatry. *Journal of Clinical Psychiatry* **67** (12) 1954–1967.

42   Martins JG (2009) EPA but not DHA appears to be responsible for the efficacy of omega-3 long chain polyunsaturated fatty acid supplementation in depression: evidence from a meta-analysis of randomized controlled trials. *Journal of the American College of Nutrition* **28** (5) 525–542.

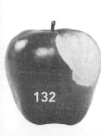

significantly better than a placebo in alleviating depressive symptoms.[43] Similarly, in borderline personality disorder (involving traits and symptoms similar to those of bipolar disorder, but in milder form), 2g a day of pure EPA reduced both aggressive and depressive symptoms.[44]

Post-traumatic stress disorder (PTSD)

Post-traumatic stress disorder (PTSD) is one of the conditions most closely linked with substance use disorders and while there has been relatively little investigation of essential fatty acids in this very heterogeneous condition, preliminary evidence from a randomised controlled trial involving 140 patients indicates that supplementation might actually help to prevent accident-related PTSD if provided immediately after the trauma.[45] The rationale for this treatment study was that omega-3 fats are known to promote neurogenesis (growth of new brain cells) in the hippocampus and that this might help to promote clearance of 'fear' memory in accident victims. The same mechanism may also be a contributory factor in the benefits reported from omega-3 supplementation for depression.

Schizophrenia

Case studies and some early trials of omega-3 supplementation for schizophrenia seemed promising, but the best results were seen in acute or first-episode patients, rather than patients who had already been chronically ill for many years. Thus, the overall evidence for omega-3 LC-PUFA as a treatment for schizophrenia remains limited and inconclusive.[46] The American Psychiatric Association noted this in their review but still recommended at least 1g per day of EPA and DHA for patients with psychosis because of the physical health benefits.[47]

43   Montgomery P & Richardson AJ (2008) Omega-3 fatty acids for bipolar disorder. *Cochrane Database of Systematic Reviews* **16** (2) CD005169.

44   Zanarini MC & Frankenburg FR (2003) Omega-3 Fatty acid treatment of women with borderline personality disorder: a double-blind, placebo-controlled pilot study. *American Journal of Psychiatry* **160** 167–169.

45   Matsuoka Y (2011) Clearance of fear memory from the hippocampus through neurogenesis by omega-3 fatty acids: a novel preventive strategy for posttraumatic stress disorder? *Biopsychosocial Medicine* **5** 3.

46   Joy CB, Mumby-Croft R & Joy LA (2006) Polyunsaturated fatty acid supplementation for schizophrenia. *Cochrane Database of Systematic Reviews* **19** (3) CD001257.

47   Freeman MP, Hibbeln JR, Wisner KL, Davis JM, Mischoulon D, Peet M, Keck PE Jr, Marangell LB, Richardson AJ, Lake J & Stoll AL (2006) Omega-3 fatty acids: evidence basis for treatment and future research in psychiatry. *Journal of Clinical Psychiatry* **67** (12) 1954–67.

Much more promising results have come from trials of EPA/DHA for the *prevention* of psychosis in so-called 'high-risk' individuals (ie. young people with a strong family history, traits associated with psychosis, and/ or transient episodes of psychotic symptoms). Pilot studies had indicated benefits in this group and a recent randomised controlled trial found that just 12 weeks of treatment with 1.2g per day of EPA/DHA could help to prevent the transition to psychosis over a 12-month follow-up period.[48] Remarkably, only four patients needed to be treated for one of them to be protected from psychotic breakdown during this time.

Implications for practitioners

■ Increasing dietary intakes of omega-3 relative to omega-6 fats in populations consuming modern diets may have benefits for a wide range of mental health conditions associated with substance use and dependence.

■ Scientific experts recommend an intake of 500mg per day of the long chain omega-3 (EPA and DHA) for general population cardiovascular health. They also emphasise that the shorter chain omega-3 (ALA) is not an effective substitute at any dose.

■ For depression and other serious psychiatric disorders, the American Psychiatric Association's treatment recommendation is at least 1,000mg per day of EPA and DHA in addition to standard treatment (*not* as a substitute).

■ This kind of intake can be achieved by eating fish and seafood several times a week, although precise omega-3 content varies by type of fish and preparation methods. Reducing dietary omega-6 (especially LA from vegetable oils) is also important in improving the omega-3/omega-6 balance.

Nutrition is fundamental to mental as well as physical health so it makes sense for dietary issues to be considered in all patients, whatever their main presenting problems. Patients with addictive disorders, and particularly with substance use and dependence, tend to have particularly poor diets and chaotic lifestyles, so that 'Type B' malnutrition (involving deficiencies in essential micronutrients) is an almost inevitable consequence of these conditions. It may also be a significant causal factor because there is ample evidence that a lack of certain essential micronutrients, including omega-3 fatty acids in particular, can disrupt mood, behaviour and cognition in many

48   Amminger GP, Schäfer MR, Papageorgiou K, Klier CM, Cotton SM, Harrigan SM, Mackinnon A, McGorry PD & Berger GE (2010) Long-chain omega-3 fatty acids for indicated prevention of psychotic disorders: a randomized, placebo-controlled trial. *Archives of General Psychiatry* **67** (2) 14–154.

ways that will exacerbate emotional problems, promote impulsivity, and impair decision-making and planning.

Current approaches to the management of substance use disorders have a very low success rate. The extremely high costs of these disorders to society as whole, as well as to those directly affected, makes a compelling case for considering any approaches that might improve outcomes without incurring significant side effects.

Attention to all aspects of diet is important in addictive disorders, as emphasised in other chapters. Relative omega-3 deficiencies are almost universal in modern developed societies, however, and the available evidence suggests that increasing dietary intakes of omega-3 (particularly the long-chain forms, EPA and DHA) could reduce the burden of a wide range of mental health conditions associated with substance use and dependence.

The evidence for benefits from long chain omega-3 (EPA and DHA) in the management of psychiatric disorders currently appears strongest for conditions involving disturbances of mood, anxiety and/or impulse control. As we have seen, these are key features of substance use and other addictive disorders, with which these conditions are strongly associated. Further studies of omega-3 supplementation in these conditions are still needed, but ensuring an adequate intake of long chain omega-3 already makes sense on general health grounds.

Omega-3: How much is enough?

Dietary intakes

At least 500mg per day of EPA and DHA is recommended for the general population to maintain cardiovascular health.[49] At least 1,000mg per day of EPA and DHA is recommended for depression and other psychiatric disorders by the American Psychiatric Association, but this is in addition to standard treatment, not as a substitute.[50]

---

49   The International Society for the Study of Fatty Acids and Lipids (2009) ISSFAL Policy Statements. See www.issfal.org.

50   Freeman MP, Hibbeln JR, Wisner KL, Davis JM, Mischoulon D, Peet M, Keck PE Jr, Marangell LB, Richardson AJ, Lake J & Stoll AL (2006) Omega-3 fatty acids: evidence basis for treatment and future research in psychiatry. *Journal of Clinical Psychiatry* **67** (12) 1954–1967.

It is possible to achieve these kinds of intakes by eating several portions of fish and seafood each week. However, the omega-3 content varies according to the type of fish and how it is prepared. Oily fish (such as mackerel, herring, sardines, pilchards, salmon or tuna) is the richest source, but any fish or seafood will make a valuable contribution to the diet. Cooking reduces the omega-3 content (and deep-frying fish in omega-6 rich vegetable oils may negate or even abolish the benefits), so light baking, broiling or grilling is preferable. Sushi, smoked salmon or other uncooked fish retain the highest omega-3 content.

Other evidence indicates that around 1,000mg per day or more may be necessary for optimal mental health, although dietary needs for omega-3 HUFA depend on the background diet, and particularly on the intake of omega-6 fats, which compete with omega-3 (both for conversion and in many of their effects on brain and body functions).[51]

Population studies indicate that for maximum protection against the degenerative physical and mental health disorders now plaguing developed countries, long chain omega-3 should make up at least 60–70% of the HUFA content of brain and body tissues. Fatty acid status can now be reliably (and cheaply) assessed from a fingerprick blood sample; and results from studies using either this method or venous samples show that the proportion of omega-3 in HUFA in populations eating modern, western-type diets is closer to 20–30%, thus indicating that there is huge room for improvement.[52]

Meaningful increases in omega-3 status (and omega-6/omega-3 balance) can best be achieved by the following kinds of dietary changes:

■ **Cut consumption of vegetable oils rich in short-chain omega-6.**

The short chain omega-6 LA is found in almost all vegetable oils and spreads, and also in the many processed foods that contain these (see Box 6.2).

Reducing the dietary intake of LA from the current 8–10% of total calories found in average US and UK diets to around 2% would effectively double tissue levels of the long chain omega-3 (EPA and DHA). This is because LA and ALA compete for the enzymes involved in synthesising long chain omega-6 and omega-3 respectively.

51 Hibbeln JR, Nieminen LRG, Blasbalg TL, Riggs JA & Lands WEM (2006) Healthy intakes of n-3 and n-6 fatty acids: estimations considering worldwide diversity. *American Journal of Clinical Nutrition* **83** 1483–1493.
52 Bell JG, Mackinlay EE, Dick JR, Younger I & Lands B (2011) Using a fingertip whole blood sample for rapid fatty acid measurement: method validation and correlation with erythrocyte polar lipid compositions. *British Journal of Nutrition* in press.

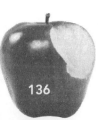

Limiting intakes of highly processed foods and snacks is crucial to reducing the excess of omega-6/omega-3 provided by most people's diets. This is, of course, particularly challenging for substance users and many others with mental health problems, as they tend to rely on these foods as a cheap source of energy.

Another reason to avoid these foods is that many contain harmful trans fats (from hydrogenated vegetable oils) for which there is no safe intake.

Box 6.2: Possible substitutes for omega-6 rich vegetable oils

- For cooking, or for salad dressings, **olive oil** (rich in monounsaturates) is an excellent substitute for most omega-6 rich vegetable oils such as corn, sunflower or safflower oils.

- **Rapeseed oil** (canola) is another alternative as it has a little ALA (but it has even more LA, so will not reduce the overall omega-6/omega-3 ratio).

- For salad dressings, **flax oil** in particular, but also walnut oil, hemp or pumpkin seed oil contain useful amounts of ALA (although cost or palatability may be an issue).

  These oils should not be used for frying or roasting as heat damages them (as it does all PUFA – but the omega-3 are more vulnerable than omega-6). Exposure to light and air also induces oxidation, so these kinds of oils also need to be kept carefully and used fairly rapidly before they become rancid.

- For frying or roasting, the much-demonised **saturated fats** (as found in butter, lard, goose fat or coconut oils) are better choices than any vegetable oils for cooking if the aim is to reduce the omega-6/omega-3 ratio.

  They are also very stable, even at high temperatures, palatable and (at least in the case of lard) cheap. Consumers can be reassured that there has never been any good evidence that saturated fats *per se* increase the risk of heart disease or other health problems when consumed in moderation.

■ **Limit consumption of meat, eggs and dairy products (rich in long-chain omega-6).**

These foods are the major dietary sources of pre-formed arachidonic acid (AA) – the key longer-chain omega-6 HUFA. An excess of AA relative to EPA and DHA promotes inflammation and increases the risk of thrombosis (blood clots), as well as disrupting the normal balance of many hormones and other signalling molecules.

■ **Increase dietary intakes of fish and seafood.**

These make an invaluable contribution to the diet, being almost the only natural food sources of the long-chain omega-3 EPA and DHA. In addition, fish and seafood are a good source of other essential micronutrients that are often relatively lacking from diets in the UK – notably selenium, iodine, zinc and vitamin D. Official dietary advice to restrict fish intake owing to concerns about possible contaminants failed to consider the potential benefits from omega-3, and appears to have been misguided, especially with respect to pregnant mothers. In a large and well-controlled birth cohort study, better developmental outcomes in the children, and less depression in the mothers, were found when the current guidelines (two portions of fish per week) were exceeded.[53,54]

Clearly, most patients with substance use disorders or other serious mental health conditions are likely to find it difficult to make healthy dietary choices without considerable support (and often practical assistance with shopping and cooking if this is feasible at all). The guidelines given here may, however, help carers and professionals to improve what is otherwise likely to be an unhealthy dietary fat intake, and they also provide a template for improving the balance of dietary fats in foods provided to patients in institutional care.

Omega-3 supplements may, however, be a more pragmatic option than major dietary changes – at least in the short-term – and in some cases prescription of these may be justifiable on physical health grounds, along

53   Hibbeln JR, Davis JM, Steer C, Emmett P, Rovers I, Williams C & Golding J (2007) Maternal seafood consumption in pregnancy and neurodevelopmental outcomes in childhood (ALSPAC study): an observational cohort study. *The Lancet* **369** 578–585.

54   Golding J, Steer C, Emmett P, Davis JM & Hibbeln JR (2009) High levels of depressive symptoms in pregnancy with low omega-3 fatty acid intake from fish. *Epidemiology* **20** (4) 598–603.

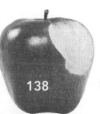

with multivitamin and mineral supplementation to redress any other micronutrient deficiencies. Ideally, nutrients are always best obtained from (natural) foods – but obtaining adequate intakes of all essential nutrients should be the priority given their fundamental importance to both mental and physical health.

Alex would like to gratefully acknowledge the Waterloo Foundation for supporting her work in this area.

Chapter 7

Allergy addiction syndrome: a plausible hypothesis?

Antony J Haynes

Introduction

The idea that you can be addicted to foods you are allergic to is highly controversial. Before exploring this idea further it is necessary to clarify some of the technical terminology involved. A food allergy is defined as an adverse health effect arising from a specific immune response that occurs reproducibly on exposure to a given food. There are various different ways of describing an adverse reaction to a food – food allergy, food intolerance, food sensitivity or hypersensitivity. The current classifications for these terms, with the speed of reactivity indicated, are as follows:

- food allergy – immediate, IgE mediated reactions
- food intolerance – delayed, mainly IgG mediated reactions
- food sensitivity – may be synonymous with intolerance, but also may exclude immune reactivity such as reactions to certain chemicals or due to maldigestion.

Note: Some American authors refer to food sensitivity as an immune mediated reaction and food intolerance as a consequence of maldigestion, as in lactose intolerance which is due to the lack of the digestive enzyme lactase.

Immunoglobulin E (IgE) responses

An IgE mediated response involves a fast-acting immunoglobulin, of which there are five: A, M, G, D and E. IgE can specifically recognise an 'allergen' – such as pollen or cat dander – and can last a lifetime once present.

IgE prompts basophils and mast cells to release mediating inflammatory chemicals (eg. histamine and leukotrienes), which cause many of the symptoms associated with allergy. These include airway constriction in asthma, local skin inflammation in eczema and increased mucus secretion in allergic rhinitis. It is presumed that this allows other immune cells to gain access to tissues. However, this can lead to a potentially fatal drop in blood pressure, as in anaphylaxis.

IgE was discovered in 1966 by the Japanese scientists Teruka and Kimishige Ishizaka[1].

Immunoglobulin G (IgG) responses

IgG are antibody molecules, each of which is composed of four peptide chains. Each has two antigen binding sites. An IgG mediated response involves a slower-acting secondary immune response. Unlike an immediate reaction, this response can lead to a manifestation of signs and symptoms up to 48 hours (or sometimes even longer) after exposure to the offending antigen.

IgG constitutes 75% of serum immunoglobulins in humans and they are made and secreted by plasma B cells.

Current terminology by immunologists refers to IgE mediated allergy as 'true food allergy'. It is generally understood that food intolerances are elicited by an IgG mediated immune response.

Terminology

For the purposes of this chapter and to both simplify matters and return to the original term, which simply means an adverse reaction to a food or substance, the term 'food allergy' will be used to include all of the above terms. The term 'allergy' in this chapter is therefore more 'broad' than the currently accepted term. However, it is relevant to note that individuals are significantly more likely to become 'addicted' to a food with a delayed adverse effect than an immediate one. It is not known if there are any addictive characteristics related to IgE food allergy.

---

1   Ishizaka K, Ishizaka T & Hornbrook MM (1966) Physico-chemical properties of human reaginic antibody. IV. Presence of a unique immunoglobulin as a carrier of reaginic activity. *Journal of Immunology* **97** (1) 75–85.

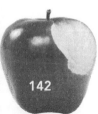

Definition of addiction

'Addiction' has been defined as physical and psychological dependence on psychoactive substances (eg. alcohol, tobacco, heroin and other drugs), which cross the blood–brain barrier once ingested, temporarily altering the chemical milieu of the brain. Once the addictive substance is reduced or stopped, withdrawal symptoms occur. [2]

Addiction can also be viewed as a continued involvement with a substance or activity despite the negative consequences associated with it. Pleasure and enjoyment of some kind need to have been originally gained. However, over a period of time involvement with the substance or activity is required simply to feel normal, as opposed to getting 'high'. This is an important distinction.

Most common causes of food allergy

Allergies are on the increase and this, in itself, is a complex topic requiring significantly more lengthy explanation. In order to provide a simple understanding, the most common reasons why someone has or develops a food allergy are listed in Box 7.1.[3]

Box 7.1: Common reasons for allergy

- High dose and repetitive consumption of similar foods
- Food additives, preservatives, food colouring agents, flavour enhancers
- Maldigestion (low stomach acid/low pancreatic enzymes)
- Imbalanced gut ecology, overgrowth of yeast, bacteria or parasites
- Antibiotic/drug therapy
- Compromised gut immunity and improved hygiene
- Excess stress
- Genetic predisposition

2   American Psychiatric Association (2000) *Diagnostic and Statistical Manual (4th Text Revision)* (TR). Washington DC: APA.
3   Haynes AJ (2005) *The Food Intolerance Bible*. London: Harper Collins.

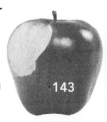

Challenging to prove

There is speculation that certain individuals are also addicted to the foods to which they have an allergy, but it is currently very challenging to prove this using the scientific methodology available. The main reason for this is that the analysis of neurotransmitters, opiate and endorphin receptors in the brain often requires brain biopsy work. The method by which it is believed that those addicted to foods may also have an allergy has so far been examined through observational science combined with an understanding of biochemistry.

Pioneers of the identification of food allergy

Historically, proponents of these observations include Herbert Leon Newbold, Theron Randolph, Marshall Mandell, William Philpott, and Dan O'Banion. (The resources section at the end of the chapter provides more information about their work.) It was observed, and then recognised, by these and other medical doctors in the mid 20th century, that the foods which provoked intolerance reactions were also the foods to which the same people had an addiction. The patients would crave the foods that elicited negative reactions (but did not provoke immediate reactivity) a number of hours later, and even as long as 72 hours after consumption. At that time, there were no scientific tests to determine the mechanism of this association and the doctors applied careful, practical, clinical trials to confirm their findings.

In the 21st century many clinicians involved in dietary therapy have observed the phenomenon of addiction to the foods to which a patient has an intolerance, and furthermore, the development of intolerance to foods which are regularly consumed in larger amounts. However, there are no conclusive studies that have examined this subject which provide a clear confirmation, even from an observational perspective. At the time of writing, exact mechanisms have not been confirmed with robust, modern scientific studies and trials.

However, in his co-authored book,[4] Jonathon Brostoff proposed a theory for food allergy addiction. He stated that immune complexes act like endorphins and stimulate their receptors – but with a key difference. These

---

4   Brostoff J & Gamlin L (1990) *The Complete Guide to Food Allergy and Intolerance*. London: Bloomsbury.

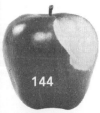

food complexes, which have been termed 'exorphins', initially stimulate the receptors by providing a sensation of reward, but they consequently blunt the opiate receptor to neurotransmitters and exorphins,[5] leading to a sensation of 'lack', thereby increasing cravings for the food. It is the desire to feel 'normal' that leads the person to seek out the foods again and again, resulting in over-consumption. As there is no immediate negative symptomology, the 'addiction' remains hidden. In this way, food allergy may comply with the definition of addiction quoted previously, in susceptible individuals.

Immunological antigen exorphin theory

It would appear that people who are more prone to addiction of any kind are more likely to have an addiction to a food and at the same time, have an allergy to that food.

The immunological antigen exorphin theory may offer an explanation behind the seemingly putative and somewhat biologically 'perverse' relationship between intolerance and addiction.

Exorphins are peptide in nature, which means they are formed by the partial digestion of proteins. As the name implies, they act rather like a weak dose of morphine. Similar to morphine, they cause addiction as well as a peculiar dreamy, euphoric feeling, which patients describe as 'being like an onlooker'. Exorphins are found in wheat and other grains, as well as milk and soya. People with robust digestive systems can digest the proteins completely and do not tend to suffer, but those with weak digestion – including low stomach acid or lack of pancreatic enzymes – break down the proteins only partly, allowing longer chains of amino acids, (ie. the exorphin peptides) to gain access to the circulation from the intestine.

Wheat is a rich source of exorphins and is eaten daily by most British people in the form of bread, biscuits, cake, pastry and pasta, not to mention less obvious sources found in foods such as sausages and soya sauce. Exorphins are ubiquitous and extremely difficult to avoid. With the ever-increasing awareness of gluten sensitivity and coeliac disease, which is estimated to affect as many as 1 in 100 people in the UK,[6] the significant presence of problems associated with gluten in the British diet is becoming

5   Zioudrou C, Streaty A & Klee WA (1979) Opiod peptides derived from food proteins: the exorphins. The *Journal of Biological Chemistry* **254** (7) 2446–2449.

6   Coeliac UK (2011) Coeliac Society website [online]. Available at: http://www.coeliac.org.uk/ (accessed July 2011).

increasingly recognised. As a result, the availability of gluten-free foods in the UK has never been so great. However, bread has the fascinating property of being virtually invisible; so habituated are people to bread that they often fail to notice its presence in a meal.

When consuming exorphins from wheat, a susceptible individual may become addicted as their innate endorphins are unable to connect to the opiate receptors. This creates a sense of need, which is met by consuming more of the particular food containing the exorphins. Interestingly, bread is the one food patients tend to forget when recalling what they ate the previous day.

The nature of cravings

It was Dr Herbert Leon Newbold who stated that *'physical addictive cravings are some of the most powerful forces that exist'*.[7] He maintained that food intolerance may occur without addiction but generally addiction is always accompanied by allergy. *'When the desire to spree-eat (hunger due to allergy or addiction) hits, it's like being struck by a freight train. You know you've been hit by a compelling force that's bigger than you are.'* [7] For this reason, it is almost always a challenge to correct the over-eating of foods in patients, quite apart from any additional emotional connections.

Allergy addiction syndrome

People who are much more susceptible to 'allergy addiction' are those who are prone to addiction, suggesting a neurotransmitter involvement. Equally, the addiction-prone person tends to have an allergic history. In this way, allergy or allergy-like sensitivities nearly always accompany addiction. For example, alcoholics are often found to be allergic to either the grains or yeast from which their favourite whiskey is brewed. The most dedicated coffee drinkers may be allergic to the coffee bean or man-made chemicals used in its production and smokers are always allergic to one or more components of cigarette smoke.

---

7   Newbold HL (1979) *Dr Newbold's Revolutionary New Discovery about Weight Loss*. New York: Rawson Associates Publishers.

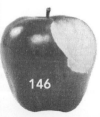

Food allergy addiction is potentially the most insidious type of allergy. It is rarely suspected because instead of causing an immediate adverse reaction, the person experiences a positive effect. Only later does a negative reaction of some kind manifest. Just as coffee drinkers may need a lift in the morning, those allergic to wheat, orange juice or sugar will get the kind of allergic-addictive pick-me-up from their addictive foods. The phrase 'allergy addiction syndrome' has been used to describe this phenomenon.

However, the relationship between allergy and addiction is often missed because the allergic side of the addiction (the symptoms of allergy) is frequently delayed.

An addicted culture?

Addiction prone individuals, because of their basic physiological makeup, are more likely to have the tendency to increase the use of cigarettes, coffee, milk, wheat or other common foods to derive a stimulatory effect. Any subtle signalling of withdrawal triggers the individual to eat the necessary food or have a cigarette, therefore the increasingly addictive nature of these substances continues in a vicious cycle.

At some point in this cycle subtle behavioural changes may be observed that can show the clinician that an addictive cycle has been established. Many aspects of modern culture – including anything which gives an immediate, short-term reward – encourage us towards addictive behaviour. Consider the easy accessibility of coffee, sweets and breakfast cereals and the amount of money spent on advertising them. These products are constantly forced into our perception. Our work culture has even incorporated the 'coffee break' so that coffee may be used frequently during the day. At the same time, this break also opens the opportunity for the consumption of other addictive substances such as caffeine, nicotine, sugar and wheat.

Allergy addiction starts young

Children can become 'cranky' unless they get their sweets or bread 'fix', which may well be more to do with blood sugar balance. Parents quickly recognise that some foods will pacify their restless infant and from the very start of their life food is used to control behaviour.

The issue becomes more complicated when one starts to consider food allergy as addiction because people will use a variety of substances, or the same substances in different forms. When an individual forces themself to give up one substance, alcohol for example, they may dramatically increase consumption of coffee, cigarettes and other addictive foods to compensate. In this way, the stimulated state is maintained and withdrawal symptoms are avoided. Only when the regular consumption of addictive substances ceases can a symptom-free state be established.

Practical testing

The best testing procedure involves a single food rotation diet where the same food is not eaten again until a full four-day period has elapsed. Some people may require a longer avoidance period. There are a number of books available on the subject of a rotation diet, even if they are not specifically aimed at those with addiction. These are detailed in the resources section.

Note: It is imperative that if an immediate-type food allergy is involved you do not engage in self-testing and instead seek advice from your doctor. This is to avoid a potentially more profound adverse reaction when reintroducing the food.

Avoidance

During the avoidance period, withdrawal and addictive cravings will be experienced and this is a very strong confirmation of the addiction. In this way, it may take a few days of avoiding a food to learn whether there is an addiction or not, dismissing all speculation about the possibilities of its existence. Most importantly, if educated about the matter this process confirms to the individual the presence of addiction. Rather than being a cause to stop the process, it is often the very thing that convinces a patient that they are on an appropriate path to better health.

Over the past 20 years, the author has conducted over 1,000 short-term avoidance trials. In virtually every case the person has come to learn about their addiction and alter their attitude to the specific food or foods, and as a consequence make improvements in their health. The strength of the

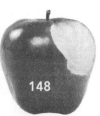

addiction has varied tremendously. Some are similar to the typical craving for coffee while others have been remarkably strong, as Newbold identified. The withdrawal symptoms can be reduced and eliminated with nutritional therapy. There are various nutrients which can help to reduce cravings and this includes vitamin C, calcium and the nutrients involved in calcium metabolism.

Following a four-day avoidance period the body most often regains its normal ability to discriminate an allergen from an addictive substance and an immediate allergic reaction will tend to ensue after eating the culprit food. This convinces most sceptics that they are allergic to their favourite food. The severity of this acute reaction is typically minor. Sometimes, the avoidance needs to be of longer duration to elicit a clear reaction.

The four-day clearing period is sufficient for the body to regain its 'unmasked' state for most foods. Hereafter, it is essential to be more aware of the addictive potential of foods or drugs consumed on a daily basis, in case they replace the food being avoided.

How do you know you have a food allergy?

If you have an addiction then it may be of value to rule out that you also have food allergy. This can be done using a food intolerance questionnaire that provides a list of symptoms and signs associated with food allergy, of the delayed type. The final part of this chapter is dedicated to the most straightforward steps that can be taken to address the allergy addiction cycle.

The Food Intolerance Questionnaire[8] from *The Food Intolerance Bible* is a good questionnaire to use when assessing whether you have a food allergy. The more of the symptoms and signs you experience on a regular basis, the more likely there is to be an allergy and the higher your score will be. When taken together with a detailed case history, a questionnaire can be a useful gauge of the presence of allergy. The frequency of consumption or desire to consume the food will reveal the addictive nature of the food(s) because it is not possible to be addicted to a food only consumed once a month.

---

8   The Food Intolerance Questionnaire can be viewed at www.foodintolerancebible.com/products/Food_Intolerance.html

Repeating a questionnaire each month will reveal whether you are being successful in addressing the food allergy and it is recommended that you keep a diary to note the severity of cravings, physical or other cognitive-related symptoms.

Nutrients vs. addiction

Although the process of avoiding foods to which one has an allergy may inevitably bring a degree of withdrawal effects, it may be possible to diminish this with the help of specific nutrients, as already mentioned.

Each person may vary in the degree of benefits conferred and it is not guaranteed. It is highly recommended to seek help from an experienced nutrition practitioner familiar with the use of the nutrients N-acetyl cysteine (NAC) and vitamin C with calcium, and its co-factors including magnesium.

N-acetyl cysteine (NAC)

NAC has a role to play in potentially helping to balance the activity of the N-methyl-D-aspartate (NMDA) receptor and glutamate receptors in the central nervous system.[9,10,11] NAC has also been shown to reduce cravings for cocaine.[12] A dose of 1,000mg twice daily on an empty stomach may be a suitable dose.

Vitamin C with calcium and magnesium

At the Haight Ashbury Clinic – a rehabilitation clinic in San Francisco – vitamin C together with calcium and its co-factor nutrients (magnesium,[13,14]

9   Hashimoto K (2009) Emerging role of glutamate in the pathophysiology of major depressive disorder. *Brain Research Reviews* **61** (2) 105–123.

10   Lavoie S, Murray MM, Deppen P, Knyazeva MG, Berk M, Boulat O, Bovet P, Bush AI, Conus P, Copolov D, Fornari E, Meuli R, Solida A, Vianin P, Cuénod M, Buclin T & Do KQ (2008) Glutathione precursor, N-acetyl-cysteine, improves mismatch negativity in schizophrenia patients. *Neuropsychopharmacology* **33** (9) 2187–2199.

11   Berk M, Jeavons S, Dean OM, Dodd S, Moss K, Gama CS & Malhi GS (2009) Nail-biting stuff? The effect of N-acetyl cysteine on nail-biting. *CNS Spectrums* **14** (7) 357–360.

12   Amen SL, Piacentine LB, Ahmad ME, Li SJ, Mantsch JR, Risinger RC & Baker DA (2011) Repeated N-acetyl cysteine reduces cocaine seeking in rodents and craving in cocaine-dependent humans. *Neuropsychopharmacology* **36** (4) 871–878.

13   Shane SR & Flink EB (1991) Magnesium deficiency in alcohol addiction and withdrawal. *Magnesium and Trace Elements* **10** (2–4): 263–268.

14   Daini S, Tonioni F, Barra A, Lai C, Lacerenza R, Sgambato A, Bria P & Cittadini A (2006) Serum magnesium profile in heroin addicts: according to psychiatric comorbidity. *Magnesium Research* **19** (3) 162–166.

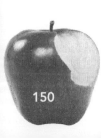

vitamins D and K, vitamin B6, potassium, boron and lysine) have been shown to reduce the cravings for drugs, including heroin.

The following ingredients comprise one formula that has been found to be effective clinically, when taken twice daily:

Vitamin C (as ascorbic scid) – 2,000mg
Vitamin D3 (as cholecalciferol) – 100 IU
Vitamin K1 (as phytonadione) – 500 mcg
Vitamin B6 (as pyridoxine hydrochloride) – 2.5mg
Calcium (85% as calcium carbonate and 15% as coral calcium) – 450mg
Magnesium (as magnesium carbonate) – 200mg
Potassium (as potassium carbonate) – 84mg
Boron (as boron citrate) – 1mg
L-Lysine – 40mg

Summary action steps

If you have addiction issues then it may be of value to consider whether you have an allergy to a certain food or foods that may contribute to your overall disposition. Although there is scepticism about its existence, you may consider this as potentially relevant. It may be worthwhile undertaking a short trial to confirm this to help achieve overall health goals (and recovery) more quickly.

1. Identify any potential culprit foods to which you may have an allergy, with the help of the Food Allergy Questionnaire. Often, it is a food consumed daily, and in abundance, such as wheat or dairy products.

2. Next, avoid the culprit food(s) for at least four days. Ensure that the food(s) are replaced with suitable alternatives prior to stopping them.

3. Observe carefully for classic withdrawal syndrome symptoms (with aggravation of existing symptoms, headaches, weakness, loss of appetite).

4. Once the withdrawal symptoms have abated, reintroduction of foods may cause immediate reactions ('unmasking'), thereby confirming the presence of allergy.

   Remember: Do not avoid and reintroduce foods which elicit an IgE immediate reaction due to potential of a magnified response requiring medical attention.

5. Consider the support of NAC and/or vitamin C, magnesium and other nutrients under supervision of an experienced and suitably qualified medical practitioner, dietician or nutritional therapist.

Hypothesis or reality?

It remains to be confirmed by modern scientific methods whether allergy addiction syndrome and the observations of some doctors and nutritional therapists over the past 60-plus years are to be determined as fact or fiction.

Further reading

Brostoff J & Gamlin L (1990) *The Complete Guide to Food Allergy and Intolerance*. London: Bloomsbury.

Haynes AJ (2005) *The Food Intolerance Bible*. London: Harper Collins.

Klee WA, Zioudrou C & Streaty RA (1978) Exorphin peptides with opioid activity isolated from wheat gluten and their possible role in the etiology of schizophrenia. In: E Usdin, WE Bunney & NS Kline [Eds] *Exorphins in Mental Health Research*. New York: MacMillan.

Mandell Dr (1988) *5-Day Allergy Relief System*. New York: Simon & Schuster.

Newbold HL (1979) *Dr. Newbold's Revolutionary New Discovery about Weight Loss*. New York: Rawson Associates Publishers.

Philpott WH (1987) *Brain Allergies*. New Canaan: Keats Publishing.

O'Banion D (1981) *15th Advanced Seminar in Clinical Ecology*. Hershey, PA: Hershey.

O'Banion D (1981) *An Ecological and Nutritional Approach to Behavioral Medicine*. Springfield Ill: Charles C Thomas.

Randolph TG (1956) Descriptive features of food addiction. *Quarterly Journal of Studies on Alcohol* **17** (2) 198–224.

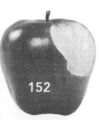

Randolph TG, Rinkel HJ & Zeller M (1950) *Food Allergy*. Springfield: Publisher.

Randolph TG (1947) Masked food allergy as a factor in the development and persistence of obesity. *Journal of Laboratory and Clinical Medicine* **32** 1547.

Rotation diet books

Edwards A & Carter J (1997) *The Rotation Diet Cookbook: 4-day plan for relieving allergies*. London: Element Books (UK).

Katahn M (1998) *The Rotation Diet*. London: Bantam

Scott-Moncrieff C (2002) *Overcoming Allergies: Home remedies, elimination and rotation diets*. London: Collins & Brown.

Chapter 8

Immunology and addiction: the potential role of the gut's mucosal immune system in promoting, treating and resolving addictive behaviours

Michael Ash

Introduction

The immune system is generally understood to be our unseen defender against infectious agents and to most people it is a complex and poorly comprehended essential in our daily life.

For simplicity of explanation, the human immune system can be divided between those components we inherit and those we acquire. The two divisions are referred to as 'innate' and 'acquired'. Each division plays a vital role in the management of our health and the resolution of infection and disease. For many years the attention in research and clinical practice was directed to the acquired part, as vaccination benefits rely on the promotion of immune memory to defend against future exposure or risk. The last 15 years has seen a significantly renewed interest in the role of the innate system and its ability to affect our health, especially in relation to non-infectious disease and illness.

The greatest concentration of both aspects of our immune system is located in the 'wet' tissues of the body. These are the thin, moist barriers that separate the outside world from our inner self, including the gastrointestinal, respiratory and genitourinary tracts, the oral and pharyngeal tissues, and the eye. Referred to as the mucosal immune system, these 'wet tissues' are under increasing scrutiny, not simply because they are common sites of infection but because they are an entry point for complex conditions involving neurological, autoimmune, cardiovascular and other seemingly diverse illnesses and loss of function.

A mass of scientific articles has appeared in the last decade depicting the immune system as an increasingly important component of key health and function deficits rather than simply as a system of defence. In particular the fields of immunology, microbiology, nutrition, epigenetics and metabolism are rapidly converging and utilising a system's biology methodology to explain our intimate relationships with the bacterial co-habitants that colonise our mucosal tissues. The way in which they co-operate appears to drive human health and also behaviour. For over 30 years data has been building to scientifically support the hypothesis that our intestinal co-habitants (bacteria, viruses and fungi) interact with macro- and micro-nutrient intakes to shape and define our immune systems from an early age.

The result is a concentrated effect created through the combination of food selection, bacterial populations and the host's health that may have 'unintended consequences' involving a wide range of dysfunction and pathologies, including addiction. This chapter will explore the emerging science that our immune system can be modified through dietary and supplemental strategies to modify its molecular messages, which may in turn assist in the management and resolution of addictive behaviour.

Note: A glossary of scientific terms can be found at the end of the chapter.

The many complexities of addiction

Addictive and associated destructive behaviours are generally seen as a reflection of an individual's choice, experiences, environment, gender, genetics and physiology. Addictive behaviour therefore results from the combination of a substance and a personality.

The brain's neuronal circuits necessary for insight, reward, motivation and social behaviours are manipulated by addiction, resulting in addicted individuals repeatedly making poor choices despite an awareness of the negative consequences. Chemicals that drive this behaviour – whether from food, sex, alcohol, drugs or other stimulants – target the brain's pleasure centres. Many addicts use the brain neurotransmitter most associated

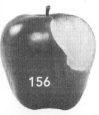

with pleasure – dopamine – as their means of pleasure promotion, however its effects on their brain is greatly enhanced by increased exposure and receptor stimulation.[1]

The consequence of repeated hedonic receptor stimulation is a loss of sensitivity, which reduces the ability to experience pleasure and results in an increased need for dopamine promotion to achieve normal levels of pleasure function (a state known as 'tolerance'). Other neurotransmitters such as glutamate can also be disturbed, leading to alterations in cognition and conditioning – a type of learning where environmental triggers promote intense cravings. Additional neurotransmitters have also been implicated in addiction, such as serotonin, gaba-aminobutyric acid (GABA) and endogenous opioids, most of which are also released from the gastrointestinal tract.

The role of the gut, its resident microbiota, the individual's overall homeostasis state (which is maintained by the constant adjustment of biochemical and physiological pathways) and the cross-communication of key behaviour modulating chemicals in the development and resolution of addictive behaviour is a novel area of cross-discipline research. It combines well with nutritional therapy proposals and supports a team approach to managing patients with behavioural and addictive problems.

To ignore the potential clinical application of the gut-based immune system, daily food selection and bacterial management, as well as the application of specialised bacterial and nutritional agents, may be to deny a powerful ally in the process of recovery. Omitting this opportunity may lead to an increased risk of intractability rather than resolution.

■ Consider the bacteria in and on your body as significant environmental triggers that are capable of reducing as well as accentuating damaging behaviours via multiple routes of immunological and other provocations.

■ The homeostatic/homeodynamic viewpoint helps to understand why there is enormous behavioural and neural variability when processing rewards between individuals.

■ The examination of human individual differences at all levels of biological and phenotypic analysis provides important insights into the mechanisms underlying complex traits. Nutritional interventions can reflect these variations and supply individualised therapy offering a personalised approach to health care.

---

1   Di Chiara G & Imperato A (1988) Drugs abused by humans preferentially increase synaptic dopamine concentrations in the mesolimbic system of freely moving rats. *Proceedings of the National Academy of Sciences* **85** 5274–5278.

What has the gut got to do with addiction?

The largest part of our innate immune system (the ancient and hard-wired (inherited) part) is in our gastrointestinal tract as this is where we determine whether something is friend or foe each time we eat and drink in a process known as 'oral tolerance'.

The cells of the innate immune system mediate inflammatory responses that are triggered through the activation of receptors on the cell surface of specialised immune defence cells; macrophages, dendritic cells, mast cells, neutrophils, eosinophils and natural killer cells. So busy are these tissues from an immunological perspective that more decisions are made in the gastrointestinal tract in a single day than the rest of our body makes in a lifetime.

It is already well established that the gut–brain immune axis – the cross communication between these two genetically rich and flexible systems (ie. the GI tract bacteria and the brain) – impacts upon animal models' brain responses. Human studies are increasingly supportive of this hypothesis.

The complex gene-to-gene interaction between genes found in gut bacteria and the brain is revealing impressive interactions. In animal models, there is a clear indication that the inter-genetic exchanges have striking effects on brain function and behaviour, including serotonin and dopamine production and attachment to receptors as well as synapse function.[2]

Do we have the guts to resolve addiction?

Yes, but we do not operate alone. As humans we share our immediate ecological environment with trillions of bacteria, fungi and viruses, many of which influence food and drug metabolism. Metabolism means the ability to absorb, distribute in the body to the site of action, detoxify and then eliminate the drug and food components (eg. via urine or bile).

2   Diaz-Heijtz R, Wang S & Anuar F (2011) Normal gut microbiota modulates brain development and behavior. *Proceedings of the National Academy of Sciences* **108** (7) 3047–3052.

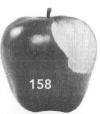

The gastrointestinal tract harbours a very impressive $>10^{14}$ microorganisms of ~40,000 species.[3] These bacteria outnumber human cells by 10 to 1 and their genetic pool is estimated to outnumber our 20,000 plus genes by over a 100 to 1. The variations in these gut microbiota ratios, relationships and tissue quality result from genetic and environmental factors such as diet, drugs, alcohol, stress, living conditions, birthplace and in utero experiences.

It is now known that individual variation in response to addictive agents is strongly influenced by the individual's biochemical and emotional state. A key and increasingly understood component of the biochemical individuality of each of us relates to the mix of bacteria – especially those in the gastrointestinal tract whose genetic code pool (microbiome), as already explained, is far greater than our own.

Individual variation in response to therapy is strongly influenced by biochemical status at the time of treatment, as reflected by metabolic phenotype, which results from the interaction of both genetic background and environmental factors including those derived from resident, transient bacteria and their food substrates. How can we harness this knowledge for the benefit of the addict?

The human microbiome: the interface between nature and nurture

A central question in psychiatry is the relative role of genes and environment in shaping behaviour. Our microbiome serves as the interface between our genes and our history of environmental exposures. Understanding and manipulating our microbiome offers the possibility of providing new insights into our neurodevelopment and our behavioural phenotypes. This dynamic affects complex processes such as inter- and intra-personal variations in cognition, personality, mood, sleep, and eating behaviour, even a variety of neuropsychiatric diseases ranging from affective disorders and addiction to autism.

Microbiomes are individualised and vary between populations and individuals with measurable consequences for addictive agent metabolism by-products. Yet

3   Frank DN & Pace NR (2008) Gastrointestinal microbiology enters the metagenomics era. *Current Opinions in Gastroenterology* **24** (1) 4–10.

very few people consider the health and function of their digestive tract and its inhabitants as being a potentially useful partner in the team approach to addiction resolution. Most attention has been directed to the brain, *not what influences the brain*, such as the gut. Perhaps it is time to think holistically and consider these tissues as a collective organ of mutual opportunity.

Our gut microbiota performs a wide range of relevant bio-transformations to addictive substances including their hydrolysis, decarboxylation, dehydroxylations, dealkylation, dehalogenation, and deamination (all mechanisms of chemical breakdown influenced by gut microbes). The dynamic interplay between bacteria and substances provides a rich source of variability in personal biochemistry and variable reactions to addictive substance ingestion, injection or inhalation. This opens up potential treatment options quite unrelated to human DNA and will require that both genetic pools are taken into consideration when looking at intervention.[4]

It is also known that gastric distress, such as dysbiosis, which is a state of altered function where gastrointestinal tissues and symbiont inhabitants are disrupted, causing an ecological shift, creates an altered homeodynamic set point.[1] Dysbiosis invokes the same stress peptides as those produced by the brain in the presence of stress and then affects the local and systemic tissues by transfer of immunomodulatory peptides to the brain via vagal nerve tissues, lymphatic systems, blood, and local inflammation.[5]

In our mucosal tissues we produce a specialised immune protein called secretory immunoglobulin A (SIgA). The abundance of IgA-secreting cells in normal mucosae means that this isotype actually comprises at least 70% of all immunoglobulins produced in humans. It is unique in that it is our only anti-inflammatory defence protein and its function and secretion depends on the colonisation of the gut with microbes. Microbe colonisation, in turn, depends on SIgA.

The output of SIgA is highly vulnerable to emotions and feelings, particularly to frustration, and is the most common immune deficiency found.[6] Using a specialised probiotic called Saccharomyces boulardi, it is

4   Wilson ID & Nicholson JK (2009) The role of gut microbiota in drug response. *Current Pharmaceutical Design* **15** (13) 1519–1523.

5   la Fleur SE, Wick EC, Idumalla PS, Grady EF & Bhargava A (2005) Role of peripheral corticotropin-releasing factor and urocortin II in intestinal inflammation and motility in terminal ileum. *Proceedings of the National Academy of Sciences* **102** 7647–7652.

6   Brandtzaeg P, Nilssen DE, Rognum TO & Thrane PS (1991) Ontogeny of the mucosal immune system and IgA deficiency. *Gastroenterology Clinic of North America* **20** 397–439.

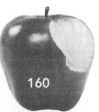

possible to encourage additional production of SIgA and aid appropriate colonisation by bacteria of the gastric tissues, and so facilitating a key component of mucosal tolerance. The result is a complex and dynamic relationship in which we are able to state that 'normal' gut microbiota are an integral part of the external environmental signals that modulate brain development, function and plasticity.[7]

Can immune-driven inflammation promote addiction?

Most people are aware of the classic signs of inflammation defined by pain, heat, redness and swelling and may be inclined to assume this chapter refers to the same. While there are similarities, the inflammation described in relation to addictive behaviour is mostly invisible to the eye, difficult to identify and ubiquitous in its locations.

Inflammation comes in many different forms and modalities and is governed by the different mechanisms of induction, regulation, and resolution. In order to comprehend the inflammation discussed here, it is easier to think of it as a low level but audible background hum that can be ignored when focused on other activities, but always returns to irritate when it is less distracted. It never goes away but varies in intensity, based on timing, location and circumstance as well as overall homeostatic health and current homeodynamic set point.

For the unfamiliar, homeodynamics is one of the basic concepts of functional medicine in which the body maintains biochemical individuality by constantly undergoing physiologic and metabolic processes. Internal and external events may alter an individual's homeodynamic set point to accommodate a defensive output of inflammatory messengers.

7   Heijtz RD, Wang S, Anuar F, Qian Y, Björkholm B, Samuelsson A, Hibberd ML, Forssberg H & Pettersson S (2011) Normal gut microbiota modulates brain development and behavior. *Proceedings of the National Academy of Sciences USA* **108** (7) 3047–3052.

Healthy inflammation is needed in the gut

In humans, the gastrointestinal tract operates best in a healthy state of low level inflammation that maintains homeostasis and keeps defences alert to invading pathogens, altered natural inhabitants and ingested foods. A mutually beneficial relationship exists here between the intestine and many of its bacterial symbionts. Symbiotic relationships can be formally categorised as mutualistic, commensal, or parasitic, although parasites are only rarely considered symbionts.

Our small intestine and colon, sometimes referred to as the 'inner tube of life', provides nutrients to our resident bacteria and in turn they aid in the digestion of food and absorption of nutrients, produce vitamins (such as biotin and vitamin K), regulate immune system function, produce essential short chain fatty acids and hinder the colonisation of pathogenic microorganisms.

Discourage unhealthy inflammation

If, however, our gastrointestinal tissues and their symbiont inhabitants are disrupted, resulting in dysbiosis, it may cause symbionts to become pathobionts. The result is a state of increased inflammation and the production of mood-altering chemicals capable of migrating away from the gut to the brain.[8] The intestinal microbiota represents a 'forgotten organ' that can execute many physiological functions, which can profoundly influence human biology, health and function.[9] Imbalances in the composition of the bacterial microbiota and health of the local tissues, known as dysbiosis, are postulated to be a significant factor in human disorders.

This increased inflammation is referred to as 'para inflammation' (para being the Greek prefix for near; as in near-to-normal).[10] The result of the dysbiosis is a change in homeostatic set points, selected initially to deal with the tissue alterations and changed to adapt to the inflammatory response. While this may be beneficial to begin with, over time para-inflammation

8   Bay-Richter C, Janelidze S, Hallberg L & Brundin L (2011) Changes in behaviour and cytokine expression upon a peripheral immune challenge. *Behavioural Brain Research* **222** (1) 193–199.

9   Dethlefsen L, McFall-Ngai M & Relman DA (2007) An ecological and evolutionary perspective on human–microbe mutualism and disease. *Nature* **449** 811–818.

10   Medzhitov R (2008) Origin and physiological roles of inflammation. *Nature* **454** (7203) 428–435.

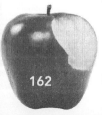

promotes maladaptation in key receptors that are often far removed from the initial trigger site and these are then perpetuated and amplified by lifestyle choices.[11] In a general sense, acute inflammation and chronic inflammation are different types of adaptive responses that are called into action when other homeostatic mechanisms are either insufficient or not competent.

These para-inflammatory responses are graded; at one extreme being close to the basal healthy homeostatic state and at the other, transitioning through altered homeodynamic states into tissue damaging inflammation. Importantly, the induction of a para-inflammatory response *does not* require overt tissue injury or infection; instead, it is switched on by tissue malfunction (such as that related to dysbiosis) and induced as a process to restore tissue functionality and homeostasis.

If tissue malfunction is present for a sustained period, para-inflammation can become chronic. It maintains a state of tissue malfunction, creating a self-perpetuating cycle of neural receptor modification that alters the receptors and the addict's hedonic homeodynamic set point, and in turn drives the addict to seek increasingly frequent exposure to their addictive substance.

Western lifestyles add to inflammatory risk

The sustained malfunction of tissues (or dysbiosis in the gut, lungs and other internal mucosal sites) can result from mutations, environmental factors or a combination. It can also be caused by the maladaptive traits responsible for modern western human diseases. Many chronic inflammatory diseases that are not caused by infection or injury are associated with conditions that were absent during the early evolution of mankind, including the continuous availability of high calorie but low nutrient density foods, a low level of physical activity, exposure to toxic and addictive compounds, complex pharmaceuticals, environmental toxins and toxicants (chemicals we produce ourselves that need neutralising by the body), drugs, persistent low levels of stress and old age.

---

11   Gluckman PD & Hanson MA (2004) Living with the past: evolution, development, and patterns of disease. *Science* **305** (5691) 1733–1736.

It is already understood that obesity and metabolic disorders (insulin resistance and hyperlipidaemia) are tightly linked to a chronic, low grade state of inflammation (elevated levels of circulating inflammatory markers such as IL-6, and C-reactive protein) and addictive behaviours.[12] It is also hypothesised that altered gut microbiota in an obese individual may contribute towards low grade inflammation, resulting in the development of metabolic diseases associated with the condition (eg. diabetes, cardiovascular disease etc.)[13] It appears that this same inflammatory milieu is capable of blunting the uptake response of immunologically sensitive neural receptors, so contributing to the increased hedonistic demands as explained above.

Brain altered by nuclear factor kappa B (NFkB) fall out

Recent animal studies have also identified that altered inflammatory responses involving the innate immune system are a key component in modifying the plasticity of brain receptors that promote addiction. In particular, a specialised immune-driven amplifying transcription factor (a protein that controls when genes are switched on or off or whether genes are transcribed or not) known as nuclear factor kappa B (NFkB) has a pivotal role to play in the promotion of immune reactive messenger chemicals, such as inflammatory cytokines, chemokines and reactive oxygen species (also called 'free radicals').

In animal models, the brain tissue genes responsible for accentuating the expression of addictive traits are increased through inflammation-induced neurogenesis (the generation of new nerve tissue). Innate immune gene induction in the frontal cortex of the brain blunts previous behavioural control, whereas it amplifies negative emotions and 'bad' feelings originating from the limbic system.[14] Inflammation enhances neural receptor plasticity and promotes addictive behaviour-related changes by promoting inflammatory cytokines and other immune messengers.

12   Kenny PJ (2011) Reward mechanisms in obesity: new insights and future directions. *Neuron* **69** (4) 664–679.

13   Cani PD, Amar J, Iglesias MA, Poggi M, Knauf C, Bastelica D, Neyrinck AM, Fava F, Tuohy KM, Chabo C, Waget A, Delmée E, Cousin B, Sulpice T, Chamontin B, Ferrières J, Tanti JF, Gibson GR, Casteilla L, Delzenne NM, Alessi MC & Burcelin R (2006) Metabolic endotoxemia initiates obesity and inulin resistance. *Diabetes* **56** 1716–1772.

14   Crews FT, Zou J & Qin L (2011) Induction of innate immune genes in brain create the neurobiology of addiction. *Brain Behaviour Immunology* **25** (1) 4–12.

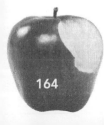

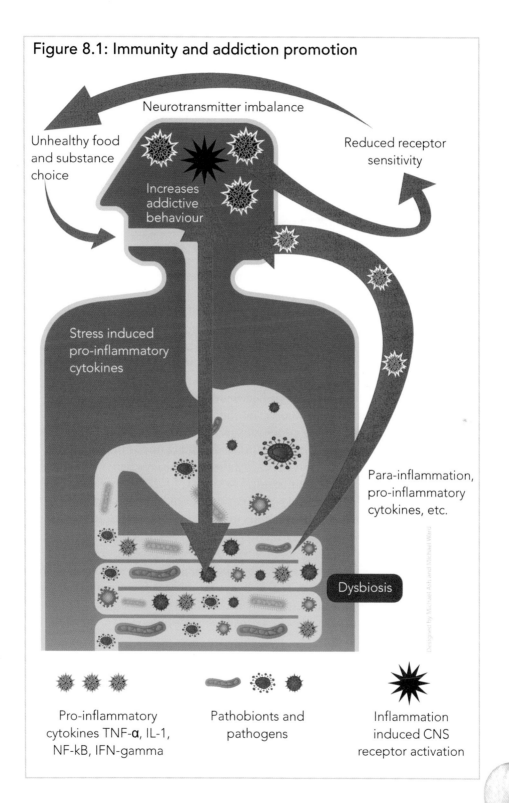

Figure 8.1: Immunity and addiction promotion

Cytokines and cell wall fragments from bacterial pathogens and pathobionts are associated with immune-related inflammation reactions and drive the development of a variety of brain-induced responses including 'sickness behaviour', which includes altered emotional behaviour, fever and changes in endocrine function. In addition, cytokines may be involved in symptoms of depressive illness, negative feelings or emotions and addictive behaviour.[15]

During the last 10 years, it has been established that pro-inflammatory cytokines induce not only symptoms of sickness, but also true major depressive disorders in physically ill patients with no previous history of mental disorders. They are now also being linked to addictive behaviour too. Immune messengers increase addictive behaviour risk and contribute to brain subjugation. In effect, the addict's brain becomes increasingly under the control of the addictive substance due to the effects of inflammatory cytokines.

Many agents are able to trigger the activation of NFkB including stress, drugs, nicotine, bacteria, viruses, yeast, sunlight, trauma, certain foods such as sugar, fat and salt (used by the food industry to promote hyperpalatability) and alcohol. Scientists have demonstrated that repeated promotion of this inflammatory cascade will mimic the progressive and persistent changes in behaviour linked to addiction and relevant neuro-degeneration. In part, this is due to the chemicals of the innate immune system, which induce anxiety-promoting, addictive behaviours. This in turn establishes or exaggerates genetic expression and changes in the brain's neurocircuitry and neurobiology that results in addictive behaviour and the setting of a new neural homeostatic set point.[16] Individual variations in sensitivity to these inflammatory changes are increasingly recognised to be attributable to in utero exposures and early life experiences, and even the immunological health of grandparents.

Remember: addiction can be defined as a primary, chronic, neurobiological disease, with genetic, psychosocial, and environmental factors influencing its development and manifestations. It is characterised by behaviours that include impaired control over drug or food use, compulsive use, continued use despite harm, and craving.

---

15 Crews FT, Bechara R, Brown LA, Guidot DM, Mandrekar P, Oak S, Qin L, Szabo G, Wheeler M & Zou J (2006) Cytokines and alcohol. *Alcoholism: Clinical & Experimental Research* **30** 720–730.

16 Breese GR, Knapp DJ, Overstreet DH, Navarro M, Wills TA & Angel RA (2008) Repeated lipopolysaccharide (LPS) or cytokine treatments sensitize ethanol withdrawal-induced anxiety-like behaviour. *Neuropsychopharmacology* **33** (4) 867–876.

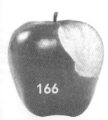

Inflammation control

If nutritional intervention is aimed at providing protection against inflammation-driven neurogenesis and protecting healthy neurogenesis, to contain negative feelings and emotions by provision of antioxidant, anti-inflammatory and antidepressant food derived substances, then additional interventions such as opiate antagonists (provided under medical supervision such as naltrexone), as well as abstinence from addictive substances, can be combined to produce a beneficial outcome. These changes link limbic affect to innate immune signalling. Therapies that positively impact on these pathways include the use of nutritional therapy in the manner explained below. The use of nutritional therapy manipulation of receptor plasticity may also impart a withdrawal symptom improvement and add to the benefits already identified using a buffered form of vitamin C (as employed by the Haight Ashbury Free Clinic in San Francisco).

Rationale for treatment

The role of the human microbiome in the predisposition, management and treatment of addictions is a novel field of discovery. The idea that the shared co-habitants of our gut are significant players in the development and resolution of addictive behaviour may seem as far-fetched as aliens controlling our minds from outer space. Yet the rapidly developing fields of psychoneuroimmunology and the exploration of the bacteria that occupy every niche in the body are revealing some fascinating insights.

As a species, we are experts at handing responsibility to others and in part this is why we have developed a mutualistic relationship with our bacteria, especially those in the gastrointestinal tract. However, we now understand that bacteria are not simply benign metabolisers of nutrients and fibres producing a few micronutrients, short chain fatty acids and various gasses. These organisms communicate constantly with the immune system, central nervous system and the delicate tissues lining the digestive tract – their resultant messages are perceived over the whole body (including the brain) either as immune tolerance or as a protest.

Pharmacologists know that our bacteria can alter medication metabolism and effects, and while the reasons for the success or failure of any clinical intervention in the treatment of addiction are manifold, a patient's pathophenotype is likely to dictate the outcome. As described, phenotypes result from many variables with genetic makeup, physiological factors such as age, gender, stress, disease, etc., and environmental factors such as diet, lifestyle, exposure to environmental toxins and environmental history (including in utero experiences), concomitant drug and alcohol usage, and even gut ecology. In this construct, addiction can be considered the result of a modular collection of genomic, proteomic, metabolomic and environmental networks that interact to yield the addictive pathophenotype.

The questions to explore are:

- Do the bacterial inhabitants of our gut influence neurotransmitters in such a way that they are manufactured more or less effectively?

- Do they alter transporter mechanisms or receptor site actions, or increase or decrease the metabolic breakdown of neuroactive peptides linked to addictive behaviour, such as dopamine?

- Do single drug usages change these bacterial relations and so increase addictive behaviour including the attraction for sugar, alcohol and psychoactive drugs? Or is it lifestyle that makes a person migrate towards a bacterial/human 'superorganism' community that favours neurotransmitter aberrations?

- If looking to assist someone to recover from addiction, is there any clinical merit in considering an approach that includes manipulating these organisms, and if so – what might one reasonably do?

Food management affects immune outcomes

It has been shown that the simple act of reducing the intake of food, either by fasting or by caloric restriction, and changing the composition of the food macro ingredients has a direct effect on the production of inflammatory cytokines, moving them towards an anti-inflammatory bias.[17]

Changing the diet to include a lower level of saturated and hydrogenated fats also reduces inflammatory cytokine output, and diets high in fats (not essential fatty acids, such as those found in fish) promote inflammatory

---

17 Macdonald L, Radler M, Paolini AG, Kent S (2011) Calorie restriction attenuates LPS-induced sickness behavior and shifts hypothalamic signaling pathways to an anti-inflammatory bias. *American Journal of Physiology: Regulatory, Integrative and Comparative Physiology* **301** (1) 172–184.

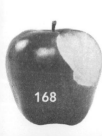

cytokine promotion, which is further aggravated by the same messengers being released from excess adipose tissues.[18]

Even when the triggers have been removed, these messengers have considerable longevity as once peripheral cytokines have been released and are bound to brain receptors, the brain remains sensitised to reactivation, promoting a fast return to behaviourally modifying immune challenges and a return to addictive behaviour.[19] Therefore, food and bacterial management needs to be seen as a long-term management strategy rather than as a single intervention. Animal studies have indicated that these receptors may be sensitised six months after the last provocation, and possibly longer.

Where necessary, this will also require body mass reduction (weight loss and increased muscle mass) as the association of numerous diseases including diabetes mellitus, heart disease, as well as depression with chronic low grade inflammation due to abdominal obesity has been confirmed. This has raised the possibility that obesity-associated inflammation affecting the brain may promote addictive behaviours, leading to a self-perpetuating cycle that may affect not only foods but addictions to drugs, alcohol, and gambling.[20] Although many addicts are very poorly nourished, significant inflammatory effects are still promoted through food selection and lifestyle, which will include nutrient deficiencies and nutrient uptake inhibition.

Increased dysbiotic immune activation has shown a prolonging effect on voluntary alcohol intake in mice and may suggest a mechanism that promotes addictive behaviours in humans.[21]

In an animal study, the researchers were surprised to see that after changing the mouse diet to one that reflected a typical westernised diet, gene expressions changed in just 24 hours. After just one day mice showed changes in their microbial composition, metabolic pathways and gene expression, and within two weeks they had developed higher concentrations of body fat.[22]

---

18   Lavin DN, Joesting JJ, Chiu GS, Moon ML, Meng J, Dilger RN & Freund GG (2011) Fasting induces an anti-inflammatory effect on the neuroimmune system which a high-fat diet prevents. *Obesity* **19** (8) 1586–1594.

19   Bay-Richter C, Janelidze S, Hallberg L & Brundin L (2011) Changes in behaviour and cytokine expression upon a peripheral immune challenge. *Behavioural Brain Research* **222** (1)193–199.

20   Heber D & Carpenter CL (2011) Addictive genes and the relationship to obesity and inflammation. *Molecular Neurobiology* (in press).

21   Blednov YA, Benavidez JM, Geil C, Perra S, Morikawa H &Harris RA (2011) Activation of inflammatory signaling by lipopolysaccharide produces a prolonged increase of voluntary alcohol intake in mice. *Brain, Behaviour, and Immunity* **25** (1) 92–105.

22   Maslowski KM & Mackay CR (2011) Diet, gut microbiota and immune responses. *Nature Immunology* **12** (1) 5–9.

Common lifestyle changes such as using a sugar replacement – often promoted as a positive lifestyle change – was shown over a three-month period of ingestion to alter the ecology of the gut with numerous adverse effects. The artificial sweetener sucralose has demonstrated numerous adverse effects in animal models, including:

■ reduction in beneficial faecal microflora

■ increased faecal pH

■ enhanced expression levels of key detoxifying enzymes, which are known to limit the bioavailability of orally administered drugs.[23]

Another study looked at dark chocolate consumption in humans and found that the daily consumption of 40g of dark chocolate (70%) during a period of just two weeks created more beneficial effects that were sufficient to manipulate gut flora ratios, thereby allowing the host to better handle stressful events.[24]

The above examples suggest that specific dietary preferences can influence basal metabolic state and gut microbiome activity that in turn may have long-term health consequences for the host. One of the ways we may be able to use individualised strategies to accurately determine what is best for each person will be through the new science of nutrimetabonomics. This is a promising future approach for the classification of dietary responses in populations, as well as for personalised nutritional management.[25]

Dietary strategies

Food selection in terms of composition and volume should reflect the evidence so far gathered. It should contain a high level of suitable fibre to encourage the development of anti-inflammatory cytokine inducing colonic bacteria, particularly the bifidobacteria species. Restoration of this balance has been demonstrated to reduce disease severity of patients and improve

23   Abou-Donia MB, El-Masry EM, Abdel-Rahman AA, McLendon RE, Schiffman SS (2008) Splenda alters gut microflora and increases intestinal p-glycoprotein and cytochrome p-450 in male rats. *Journal of Toxicology and Environmental Health* **71** (21) 1415–1429.

24   Martin FP, Rezzi S, Peré-Trepat E, Kamlage B, Collino S, Leibold E, Kastler J, Rein D, Fay LB & Kochhar S (2009) Metabolic effects of dark chocolate consumption on energy, gut microbiota, and stress-related metabolism in free-living subjects. *Journal of Proteome Research* **8** (12) 5568–5579.

25   Rezzi S, Ramadan Z, Martin FP, Fay LB, van Bladeren P, Lindon JC, Nicholson JK & Kochhar S (2007) Human metabolic phenotypes link directly to specific dietary preferences in healthy individuals. *Journal of Proteome Research* **6** (11) 4469–4477.

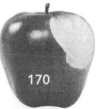

well-being in healthy volunteers.[26] Selecting foods and other agents that cause changes in the gut microbiota's composition and/or activity(ies) to strengthen symbiosis and resolve dysbiosis will induce beneficial physiological effects in the GI tract. This reduces the risk of dysbiosis and associated intestinal and systemic pathologies, in turn altering neurobiological events for the better. [27]

Some dietary fibre sources are more readily fermented by intestinal bacteria than others, impacting on physiological outcomes. One favoured fibre source is found in apples, especially when cooked, as apples modify bacterial composition and are anti-inflammatory (see recipe). Apples also help to alter the pathobiont mix of bacteria in human guts when consumed regularly; suggesting a role for their use in mild to moderate dysbiosis induced inflammation and loss of tolerance.[28] In a small but clinically interesting study, healthy adults on a diet of two apples a day for two weeks noted an increase in bifidobacteria species, an increase in lactobacillus and a decrease in dysbiotic bacteria.[29]

Root crops and legumes are also good sources of dietary fibre and produce short chain fatty acids after fibre fermentation, such as acetate, propionate and butyrate.[30] Short chain fatty acids are an essential component in the management of a tolerogenic environment in the gut and contribute to anti-inflammatory management of local as well as systemic tissues. Many people consume their fibre as wheat or other grains that contain gluten. Gluten sensitivity, while a somewhat controversial area in dietetic arenas, is increasingly recognised in scientific journals and may inadvertently add to the inflammatory milieu.[31] Gluten (mixture of proteins, including gliadins and glutelins that are found in wheat, rye, barley and possibly oats) sensitivity encompasses a collection of medical conditions in which gluten has an adverse effect.

26   Silvi S, Verdenelli MC, Orpianesi C & Cresci A (2003) EU project Crownalife: functional foods, gut microflora and healthy ageing. Isolation and identification of Lactobacillus and Bifidobacterium strains from faecal samples of elderly subjects for a possible probiotic use in functional foods. *Journal of Food Engineering* **56** 195–200.

27   Roberfroid M, Gibson GR, Hoyles L, McCartney AL, Rastall R, Rowland I, Wolvers D, Watzl B, Szajewska H, Stahl B, Guarner F, Respondek F, Whelan K, Coxam V, Davicco MJ, Léotoing L, Wittrant Y, Delzenne NM, Cani PD, Neyrinck AM & Meheust A (2010) Prebiotic effects: metabolic and health benefits. *British Journal of Nutrition* **104** (2) 1–63.

28   Chow J & Mazmanian SK (2010) A pathobiont of the microbiota balances host colonization and intestinal inflammation. *Cell Host Microbe* **7** (4) 265–276.

29   Shinohara K, Ohashi Y, Kawasumi K, Terada A & Fujisawa T (2010) Effect of apple intake on fecal microbiota and metabolites in humans. *Anaerobe* **16** (5) 510–515.

30   Trinidad TP, Mallillin AC, Loyola AS, Sagum RS & Encabo RR (2010) The potential health benefits of legumes as a good source of dietary fibre. *British Journal of Nutrition* **103** (4) 569–574.

31   Newnham ED (2011) Does gluten cause gastrointestinal symptoms in subjects without coeliac disease? *Journal of Gastroenterology and Hepatology* **26** (3) 132–134.

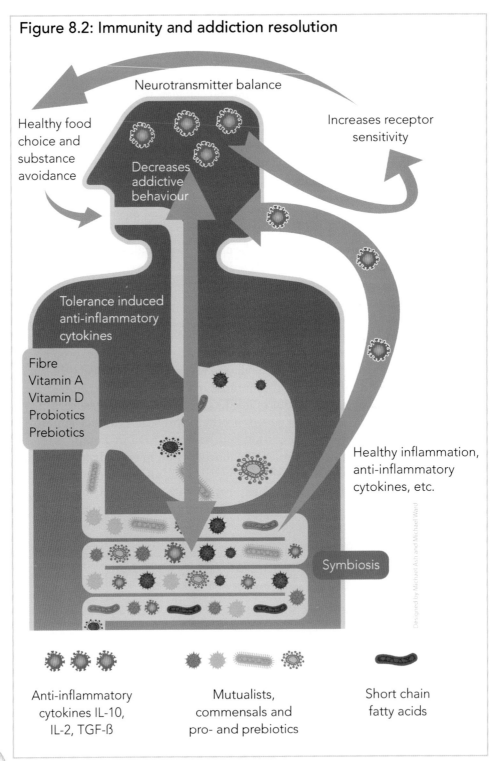

Figure 8.2: Immunity and addiction resolution

Additionally, knowledge is increasing about the microbial bioconversion of beneficial phytonutrients called polyphenols. The main dietary sources of polyphenolic compounds, which are converted into advantageous bioactive metabolites in the colon are fruits (eg. citrus fruit, apples, grapes and berries), wine, tea, soy, cacao and vegetables. With the evolving science of nutrimetabonomics, it will become increasingly easy to use foods to reduce addictive traits by manipulating food substrate bioconversion into more potent compounds with focused antioxidant and/or anti-inflammatory activity.

Key vitamins and minerals are also required to ensure mucosal tolerance and these include zinc, vitamin A and vitamin D, often found to be depleted in individuals that remain covered and living in northern hemispheres. Being of European descent also confers a unique genetic risk for vitamin A insufficiency as up to 40% of northern Europeans lack a genetically coded enzyme in the gut to convert beta carotene into retinol (the active form of vitamin A), which is required to maintain mucosal immune tolerance.[32]

Dietary and supplemental suggestions

- A diet high in fibre-rich root vegetables and fruits ie. two large Bramley apples per day to alter microbial composition and favour an anti-inflammatory output through phenolic compound activation. These foods are also prebiotics.

- A broad range of micronutrients designed to meet any lifestyle or genetically determined deficiencies, in particular the fat-soluble vitamins A and D should be supplemented along with the mineral zinc. Doses for the ingredients should reflect the individual needs of the addict, but may range from vitamin A (as retinyl palmitate) 5,000 µg to 25,000 µg per day; vitamin D3 1000 µg to 10,000µg per day; zinc (as gluconate and citrate) 5mg to 25mg per day.

- Periods of food abstinence (fasting) to assist with body composition changes and to favour anti-inflammatory activity – obviously this must be undertaken in context and not be recommended for individuals where their addictive behaviour already favours food exclusion.

- The addition of strain-specific colonic bifidobacteria and small intestinal lactic acid bacteria to promote a return to a state of symbiosis.

---

32   Leung WC, Hessel S, Méplan C, Flint J, Oberhauser V, Tourniaire F, Hesketh JE, von Lintig J & Lietz G (2009) Two common single nucleotide polymorphisms in the gene encoding beta-carotene 15,15'-monoxygenase alter beta-carotene metabolism in female volunteers. *FASEB Journal* **23** (4) 1041–1053.

- The inclusion of Saccharomyces boulardii, a gastric friendly yeast, to support immune function, reduce inflammation and repair any barrier defects as well as aid in the colonisation ratio changes in commensal bacteria.

- Maintenance of regular bowel and kidney activity through optimal hydration.

- Reduction of body mass so that muscle tissue increases and adiposity decreases.

- Consider the use of buffered vitamin C as a nutrient to diminish cravings. It has strong buffering actions to offset hyperacidity associated with cell pathology. Vitamin C alone has some mild anti-addictive properties. The ascorbate form of calcium (which forms from the reaction of the calcium carbonate and ascorbates) appears to be very well absorbed. High levels of calcium with additional magnesium and potassium provide a balancing and alkalising effect.

Recipe: Stewed healing apples and immune co-factors

Ingredients for cooking

6 Bramley cooking apples (or apples of choice, preferably grown organically)

1/2 cup water

1/2 cup raisins/sultanas

2 tsp cinnamon

Directions

- Peel and core the apples and chop them into small pieces.
- Put all the ingredients into a covered, heavy-bottomed pan and cook for 15 minutes, stirring regularly.
- When cooked, the apples should be soft and no longer identifiable as apple slices. The colour should be a russet brown with the added cinnamon.

Other ingredients

- Some people will find the apples too tart. In this case, avoid adding sugar and add 1 tsp of larch arabinogalactan for sweetness. Larch arabinogalactan is a polysaccharide powder derived from the wood of the larch tree, and is a useful source of dietary fibre with potential therapeutic benefits as an immune stimulating agent.

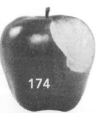

- 1 Saccharomyces boulardii 250mg capsule sprinkled on or swallowed separately. Saccharomyces boulardii is classified as a probiotic and promotes a number of beneficial changes in the gut including the increased expression of SIgA and better enzymatic breakdown of carbohydrates.
- 1 mix of Bifidobacteria (mixed strains) (500mg) 5 billion CFU (colonising forming units) sprinkled on top or swallowed separately. Bifidobacteria are important components of the lower intestine and break down foods, and modulate immunity in the gut and elsewhere.
- 1 x Lactobacillus rhamnosus (the best studied is Lactobacillus GG) sprinkled on top or swallowed separately. This bacteria is found mainly in the upper part of the digestive tract, promotes good food breakdown and supports a healthy immune response.
- ½ 150g container of organic natural yogurt (dairy) or soy equivalent.
- 6–8 blueberries and 4–5 almonds in their skins. Almonds and berries are also beneficial to the mucosal immune system.
- Finally, if required, a teaspoon of Manuka honey. This also assists with immune balance.

For additional assistance with the application of an anti-inflammatory diet, food choice and supplements, consider contacting a registered nutritional therapist.

Concluding thoughts

Based on our current understanding, humans are best described as complex biologic 'superorganisms' and interventions to modify addictive behaviours should take this model into account when planning therapeutic interventions. This includes considering and respecting the gut–brain axis and how dietary choices may either beneficially or adversely affect it.

Glossary of scientific terms

Commensals

Normally occurring species living on or within another organism, and deriving benefit without harming or benefiting the host.

Cytokines and chemokines

Small proteins released by cells that have a specific effect on the interactions between cells, on communications between cells or on the behaviour of cells. The cytokines includes the interleukins, lymphokines and cell signal molecules, such as tumour necrosis factor and the interferons, which trigger inflammation and respond to infections.

Dysbiosis

Humans are colonised by multitudes of commensal organisms representing members of five of the six kingdoms of life; however, our gastrointestinal tract provides residence to both beneficial and potentially pathogenic microorganisms. Imbalances in the composition of the bacterial microbiota is known as dysbiosis.

Genotype

This is the 'internally coded, inheritable information' carried by all living organisms. This stored information is used as a 'blueprint' or set of instructions for building and maintaining a living creature. These instructions are found within almost all cells (the 'internal' part). They are written in a coded language (the genetic code), are copied at the time of cell division or reproduction and are passed from one generation to the next ('inheritable'). These instructions are intimately involved with all aspects of the life of a cell or an organism. They control everything from the formation of protein macromolecules, to the regulation of metabolism and synthesis of enzymes.

Isotype

Any of the subclasses of immunoglobulins produced by the immune system and defined by the chemical and antigenic characteristics of their constant regions. In humans, the five human isotypes are: IgA, IgD, IgG, IgE and IgM. IgG and IgA also have subclasses.

Microbiome	Microbiome is the totality of microbes, their genetic elements (genomes), and environmental interactions in a defined environment. A defined environment could, for example, be the gut of a human being or a soil sample.
Mutualists	Originated from the Latin word *mutuus*, meaning lent, borrowed, or mutual. A relationship between two organisms where both organisms benefit. For example, bacteria that expand in the intestinal niche and provide metabolic pathways complementing the digestive functions of the host.
Neurotransmitter	A neurotransmitter is a messenger of neurologic information from one cell to another.
Nutrimetabonomics	Nutrimetabonomics is the collection and analysis of fluids and metabolites produced by a human and its microbes after eating certain foods. It assesses the food's effects on metabolism.
Pathobionts	Normally occurring species that due to changes in the environmental cues are seen as a threat by the immune system.
Parasite	Originates from the Greek words *para* and *sitos*, meaning 'beside' and 'food', or one who eats at another's table. A relationship between two organisms where one organism benefits at the expense of the other. Mostly defines the behaviour of a pathogen.
Pathophenotype	A new approach to classifying human disease that uses conventional reductionism and incorporates the non reductionist approach of systems biomedicine that takes into account the interactions of multiple systems on the human genome. Such phenotypes result from many variables with genetic makeup, physiological factors such as age, gender, stress, disease, etc., and environmental factors such as diet, lifestyle, exposure to environmental toxins and environmental history (including in utero experiences), concomitant drug and alcohol usage, and even, or perhaps especially in light of emerging experimental work in areas such as diabetes and obesity and gut microbiology.

Phenotype	This is the 'outward, physical manifestation' of the organism. These are the physical parts, the sum of the atoms, molecules, macromolecules, cells, structures, metabolism, energy utilisation, tissues, organs, reflexes and behaviours; anything that is part of the observable structure, function or behaviour of a living organism.
Proteomic	The term 'proteomics' was coined in 1994 by Marc Wilkins who defined it as *'the study of proteins, how they are modified, when and where they are expressed, how they are involved in metabolic pathways and how they interact with one another'.*[33]
Receptor	A receptor is a molecule found on the surface of cells, which receives specific chemical signals from neighbouring cells or the wider environment within an organism. These signals tell a cell to either respond, or not respond, and differ in shape and sensitivity between different tissues and systems.
Short chain fatty acids (SCFA)	Short chain fatty acids having a chain length up to roughly six carbon atoms long. They are produced by bacterial anaerobic fermentation, particularly of dietary carbohydrates, in the large intestine. They are readily absorbed and are metabolised in the liver and muscle tissues, producing energy and supporting tolerance through inflammation control.
Synapse	A synapse is a junction between two nerve cells, consisting of a minute gap across which nerve impulses (electrochemical signals) pass by diffusion of a neurotransmitter.
Symbionts	An organism in a symbiotic relationship.
Symbiosis	Originated from the Greek words *syn* and *biosis*, meaning 'with' and 'living' coined in 1879 by the mycologist Heinrich Anton de Bary. The original meaning of symbiosis is the 'living together of unlike organisms'. Symbiosis is generally understood as a relationship between two organisms from which both organisms benefit.

---

33   Wilkins M. Proteomics data mining. Expert Rev Preteomics. 2009 Dec;6(6):599-603

Chapter 9

The proof is in the pudding: a personal account of how I self-manage my addictions

Yvonne Luna

I was a sweet child. By that, I don't mean I was lovely, but that I loved sweets. Like many children, I was addicted to sugar from year dot; it literally was (and still is) in everything from baby food purées to soups and meats. I have always been moody – I had terrible tantrums all through my childhood, and continue, even now, to fly off the handle and lose control if I let my diet slip.

I had no idea diet was playing such a large part in my continuous mood swings, which threw me from nirvanic highs to abysmal lows. My drugs of choice, by which I self-medicated, were confectionaries. Even the most suicidal of depressions could be temporarily lifted by a cocktail of brightly coloured, pill-shaped sweets, two or three bars of chocolate and a tub of ice cream. As I passed through the supermarket counter with my treasures, I would joke with the till operator saying, 'Dinner…' Except it wasn't a joke: it really was my dinner. I would eat £2 or £3 worth of sweets instead of a meal. Sometimes I was too depressed to eat, but I could still eat sweets. As I never seemed to put on weight, I couldn't see any reason to change my diet – like most people, I only saw sugar as a danger to one's figure or teeth, little realising what effect it was having on my mental health. I suspected sugar contributed to my highs, but never made the equation that what goes up must come down ie. I never linked my huge intake of sugar to my recurrent depressions.

At many points in my life I contemplated using antidepressant drugs, even getting to the point of being prescribed them and collecting the prescription. But I never took them. I was holding off for something because I was sure I could find the answer to my depressions. I refused to believe there was anything wrong with me – I was born perfect, wasn't I? So what happened?

Around 2003, a book title caught my attention. I must have already been snooping around the idea that my diet might be playing a part in my depressions, which, when they weren't leading me into increasingly bizarre and destructive behaviours, were causing me to literally sleep my life away. The book was called *Potatoes, not Prozac* by Kathleen DesMaisons.[1] The title seemed to sum up my quest to avoid medication, and I started to read. Finally the chocolate penny dropped. It was to prove a life-changing book for me, as I learnt how my little white friend (ie. sugar) could act on the body and brain in a similar way to drugs and alcohol, and become addictive. Everything I read made sense, and spoke to my own personal experiences.

The first step involved analysing what I ate without changing my diet, but by keeping a food diary. In this way, I was able to see and feel the direct relationship between a skipped meal replaced by sweets, and the consequent depression as the effects of the sugar high wore off. I learnt about eating slower releasing carbohydrates, like potatoes, instead of quick-fix refined sugars. I followed the plan and discovered my mood levelled out, but not before suffering terrible withdrawal pangs, where I would literally 'see' Mars bars floating across my mind, as if to say: 'All you need to do is eat me, and all this pain will go away…'

The withdrawal pains reminded me of those I'd experienced when I gave up smoking; then, too, I had visions of cigarettes before my eyes, promising to release me from the mental and emotional anguish of the nicotine withdrawal. The similarity in symptoms furnished enough proof for me to conclude that sugar, like nicotine, was an addictive substance, rather than a food. It felt impossible to stop eating chocolate altogether, but DesMaisons' plan initially allowed the forbidden fruit to be eaten as long as you ate a full meal first, so that you ceased to see the chocolate as food, but started to see it more as a drug, like an after-meal cigar, coffee or digestif. Also, of course, I could not eat so much sugar when my body was full of proteins, vegetables and savoury carbohydrates.

Another discovery I made was that by eating a large plate of salad containing mostly lettuce with a chopped clove or two of raw garlic and fresh ginger, I could lift a depression. There seems to be research that backs up this finding, with studies suggesting that 'lettuce opium' induces a slight state of euphoria and relaxation, and apparently makes rabbits sleepy

---

1   Editor's comment: Numerous clinical accounts of sugar addiction have been published over the past decades in the self-help genre. Although the science of food addiction is still in its infancy, it has been shown that sugar-bingeing in animal models produces addictive-like behaviour that includes withdrawal syndrome.

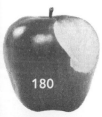

and 'chilled'. I don't understand how the raw garlic works on the brain, but again there has been research claiming that others, too, have gained emotional and mental improvements after consuming raw garlic.

I cannot pretend to be free from my sugar addiction, but I am managing it, and know that if I feel depression creeping back, I can usually halt it in its tracks by disciplining myself to cut out sugar and eat unrefined foods and salad to get back on track. One good compromise I have discovered is making my own hot chocolate out of cocoa powder (preferably raw), hot milk or soya, and a teaspoon of honey, though now I don't tend to need the honey added. To alleviate a sugar craving, this can do the trick, and prevent a full escalation into buying and devouring an entire box, or several bars of my favourite chocolates, which I know will only leave me feeling worse than ever. It has been pointed out to me that honey, too, is a kind of sugar, and, as I say, this is very much a compromise solution, but it works because of the difference in availability and cost between sugar and honey. Sugar, as I mentioned, is in nearly everything, whereas honey is not.

This method works for me for the simple reason that if I tell my brain that I can have occasional honey, but not sugar, then I am limited to a narrower choice of products, and all easily available sweets, chocolates, biscuits and cakes are out of bounds. I am mainly forced to make my own honeyed goods, which takes more care, love and consideration of what I'm doing – it removes thoughtless and mindless bingeing, where as often as not, I wouldn't even be aware of how many bars I was eating, in much the same way as I used to smoke cigarettes automatically and unconsciously. You could say that honey is my 'methadone'.

Similarly, with reference to the potatoes mentioned earlier, some people have said to me that mashed potato is 'bad' for you, pointing out that potatoes can act on the body and mind like a sugar. Even if this is the case, potato addiction could hardly become a problem: it's hard to binge on something that takes so long to cook, fills you up, and is not as readily available as sweets. DesMaisons is not advocating chips or crisps, but potatoes baked in their skins – the sheer bulk of the potato would slow you down, in much the same way as it would take longer to develop an alcohol addiction when having to consume voluminous pints of beer compared to the faster route of spirits. Besides, potatoes are actually a food: they contain protein, fibre, vitamins and more. The same cannot be said of white sugar, which contains no nutritional value whatsoever. Just because it contains calories does not make it a food; alcohol, too, contains calories, but no one would dream of putting alcohol on a food chart or considering it as food!

Now that I am making the connection between sugar and my moods, it is easier for me to cut it out, knowing what mental misery awaits me if I do indulge in this destructive habit. It does take a huge amount of discipline though – we are bombarded daily with advertisements for sugar products. I believe sugar is put into products as a way of priming our taste buds. I grew to question my favourite foods and analyse them: of course I loved tomato soup best – it's full of sugar, that's why. I can now taste the misplaced sugar in things, and no longer accept that soup is supposed to taste sugary. Traditionally, soups were sweetened with sweet vegetables, like swedes and parsnips.

Adding sugar is sheer laziness and dishonesty on the part of the producers. I am reminded of the rumour in the 1970s, that a certain cat food brand was putting heroin in its products in order to induce nine out of ten cats to prefer it, and pick out the bowl containing their brand. Are manufacturers not using a similar tactic when they lace their products with white sugar, a substance now increasingly acknowledged as being highly addictive? My own taste buds had become so sugar-accustomed that I could no longer taste the sweetness in anything else. Since cutting out refined sugars, I have been astonished to discover the natural sweetness of grapes, raisins, dates, melon, pears, oranges – all foods which before would have held no flavour for me, so dulled had my taste buds become.

The other food that seems to affect my mental health is gluten. I asked my doctor for a test to see whether gluten intolerance might be involved in my depressions, but the blood test service they offer only relates to gluten's connection to coeliac diease or Crohn's disease. According to the test results, I have no problem with wheat, despite the fact that I become depressed and deeply tired within a very short time of consuming wheat products, especially bread. So although, generally speaking, one can deduce that the proof is in the pudding, so to speak, I here find myself in a situation where my body, mind and emotions are clearly telling me one thing, while medical science is telling me another. It takes confidence to trust one's gut instincts in this case. I have to remind myself that throughout history even the kindest doctors have got things wrong. For example, my own mother was offered Thalidomide when pregnant with my brother. Like me, she trusted her intuition about things, and refused it, despite doctors' protestations that it was perfectly safe.

Another problem I have is with marketing. As a single person on a limited income, I find it hard to find single food items when products are increasingly being sold in packets of two, four, six or even a whole bag, especially in supermarkets, where the more you buy, the cheaper it gets.

Plus, the special offer displays always seem to be highlighting the products that are the worst for us: cola, biscuits, sugary cereals, chocolates and crisps. These offers appeal to our sense of greed: why go to the bakers and buy one doughnut for 60p when you can get a bag of five at a supermarket for 78p? Not to mention the depressing thought that you're not supposed to be single, when so many items are only packaged for two or more.

Also, on the point of marketing, a lot of people I've met don't seem to distinguish between real fruit juice and squash, and are, in general, all too easily fooled by deceptive imagery on labels. I laughed when I saw a bleach bottle (now mercifully removed from the supermarket shelves) sporting images of oranges on its label. This was an obvious, and dangerous, marketing fault. Yet no one seems to query fruit 'juices' that also show images of fruit, though the actual quantity of real juice present is extremely low, or even absent altogether in many 'squashes'. Again, it's all about sugar, flavouring and colouring, and nothing more.

This also applies to other products, where it seems to be legal to show pictures of happy chickens, pigs etc. on packages that contain meats produced under the worst possible farming methods. It is my belief and experience that psychological and spiritual connections to food affect mental health. I always endeavour to eat foods that are free range and organic, even if it means food shopping takes up most of my budget. Many studies have indicated that the consumption of pesticides and antibiotics used in intensive farming affect our health on a physical level, but I believe that, of equal importance, is the fact that, as intelligent beings, we are also liable to absorb misery through what we eat, when we eat something with the full awareness and knowledge of how this meal was produced.

Cheap often equates with cruelty. To produce things cheaply, we damage the environment: poisoned insects poison the birds that eat them, or simply die out, so there are insufficient insects for the birds to eat. Some people complain that organic and free range products are expensive, but they are not. They are the correct price. Rather than worrying about these products being expensive, we should be looking at how and why certain products are produced so cheaply, and be suspicious of cheap meats and other consumables. In terms of how this relates to mental health, I do not believe that we can consume products we know have been produced using cruel or irresponsible methods, and live with a good conscience. I believe we all need to eat feel-good foods the same way we need to see feel-good films.

Quite simply, I feel better about myself, and about life in general, knowing that my money (which is energy) is supporting positive experiences and practices. I believe this spiritual and moral connection between what we eat and our mental health could be flagged up a lot more. We are what we eat, so if the creatures we eat, and our natural world in general, matter, then we can believe that we, too, matter. For me, in mental health terms, this belief system goes a long way – every little helps, and each individual gesture makes a difference to one's own self-belief and esteem.

Finally, it is my belief that many westerners are obese because, paradoxically, they are starving. As they fill their stomachs with a bulk of nutrient-deficient products, which can hardly even be classified as 'food', their bodies crave nutrition: proteins, vitamins, minerals, essential fats and complex carbohydrates. As Dr Carl Pfeiffer put it in his book *Mental Illness: The nutrition connection: 'Those who are well nourished are unlikely to become addicted, or to be so attracted to addictive substances, most of which create a lift of energy, sought by the undernourished.'* Empty calories lead to addiction, and all its inherent mental health problems. I, too, have experienced the phenomenon Pfeiffer mentions of tending to crave the substances that are precisely the ones most addictive and toxic to me.

Anecdotal evidence is often scorned by many in the medical profession. I have searched for my own answers to my depressions, and while I would never be so ignorant as to claim that all my mental health problems have been caused or cured by diet, my experiences point a chocolate finger at the role certain edible substances, most notably refined sugar and gluten, have played in my mental and emotional states.

You need guts to do anything brave or merit-worthy in this life, and by filling those guts with empty calories we are prone to leading empty lives. My investigations have led me to realise the importance of other factors too: physical exercise, spirituality, friendship, and so forth. But increased awareness and knowledge about my nutritional needs and poisons has played a key role in my ability to enjoy ever improved mental health. Observing the connection between what I eat and how I feel has furnished all the proof I need of the importance of the link between food and mood. It is in certain people's interests to disbelieve that white sugar can be addictive; but there was a time when many denied cigarettes were addictive, saying similarly that there was no proof. As a teenager, people laughed at me when I said a day would come when you could buy wholemeal bread and other health foods in supermarkets and not just in specialist stores. (This was at a time when I despaired that most only stocked white bread.) Now my ambitions include seeing stricter regulations on deceptive food marketing; and yes, why not, a return of the Sugar Tax that was abolished by Gladstone in 1874. Not only would this solve a lot of health problems and make people think differently about sugar, but it might just solve the government's deficit problems to boot! I have sweet dreams, and not the sugary kind.

Drug terms

Abstinence means not using substances. The term's use varies but abstinence-based or abstinence-focused can be used to refer to drug or alcohol treatment programmes that aim to help the person stop using drugs or alcohol for the rest of their lives. The definition of abstinence varies; for example, some people do not consider an individual to be abstinent when they are in receipt of substitute prescribing such as methadone.

Addiction see dependence. The term addiction is inextricably linked to society's reaction to the user, and so medical experts try to avoid using it, preferring the term 'dependence' instead.

Addict is a term often used to describe someone who is dependent on drugs. Many people in the field prefer to talk of 'dependent drug users' instead, as 'addict' can be seen as a morally loaded term that reduces the individual to the sum of their behaviour.

Blood-borne virus (BBV) is a virus that people carry in their blood. BBVs can spread to another person, whether the carrier of the virus is ill or not and may be transmitted sexually or by direct exposure to infected blood or other body fluids contaminated with infected blood. The main BBVs of concern are: hepatitis B, hepatitis C and hepatitis D, which all cause hepatitis, a disease of the liver, and human immunodeficiency virus (HIV) which causes acquired immune deficiency syndrome (AIDS), affecting the immune system of the body.

Controlled drugs in the UK are those controlled under the Misuse of Drugs Act. This divides drugs into three classes: A, B and C according to an assessment of their danger to individuals and society at large. Class A attracts the highest penalties for possession and supply. These drugs are also controlled under the Misuse of Drugs Regulations which divides drugs into five schedules according to their medicinal value. Schedule 1 would be for drugs for which a prescription is not available such as LSD or ecstasy. Drugs like morphine, which is used in the treatment of severe pain, are in Schedule 2. The schedules cover such issues as manufacture and supply, prescribing and appropriate record-keeping.

Nutrition and Addiction: A handbook © Pavilion Publishing (Brighton) Ltd 2011

Come down	is the hangover or after-effect of taking a drug. Reflecting the low feeling experienced after the high of taking a drug, come down is mostly associated with the after effects of stimulant taking, in particular ecstasy, which can last anything up to four days.
Dependence	describes a compulsion to continue taking a drug in order to feel good or to avoid feeling bad. When this is done to avoid physical discomfort or withdrawal, it is known as physical dependence; when it has a psychological aspect (the need for stimulation or pleasure, or to escape reality) then it is known as psychological dependence.
Dependent drug user	is someone whose drug use causes serious physical, social or psychological problems for them and/or for those around them. Another frequently used term to describe this group is 'problem drug user'.
Designer drugs	is a term coined in the 1980s to describe drugs specifically synthesised to circumvent regulations on controlled substances. Ecstasy is often cited as a designer drug, but this is incorrect. As a drug which is chemically similar to amphetamine, there was no need for new legislation to control its use when it became popular. Drugs such as Spice or mephedrone could, however, be considered designer drugs. Spice was synthesised to mimic the effects of cannabis, a controlled drug, and mephedrone was developed as a stimulant that would (initially at least) circumvent the law.
Detoxification	is the process by which a user withdraws from the effects of a drug. It usually refers to withdrawal in a safe environment (a detoxification/detox unit), with help on hand to minimise the unpleasant symptoms.

Drug use/ misuse/abuse   drug use is an easy term to understand. Misuse and abuse are more difficult to pin down, as they are highly subjective. In most circles, 'misuse' means using in a socially unacceptable way. However, the definition currently being adopted defines misuse as using drugs in a way that results in experience of social, psychological, physical or legal problems related to intoxication and/or regular consumption. The term 'abuse' may be regarded as too judgemental, as it suggests impropriety regardless of how the drug is being used. As abuse and misuse can be morally 'loaded' terms, some prefer to talk of drug-taking, or of harmful or problematic use instead, when appropriate.

Harm reduction   refers to policies and projects which aim to reduce the health, social and economic harms associated with the use of drugs. Needle exchange programmes, for example, are a key harm reduction intervention. Harm reduction recognises that society is unlikely to ever be drug, drink or nicotine-free. Harm reduction does not exclude abstinence as a goal for individuals who are dependent but, rather, provides people with pragmatic choices such as limiting their intake or using drugs more safely.

Headshops   are retail outlets which sell a wide variety of paraphernalia that may be associated with the use of illegal drugs (such as pipes or herb grinders for use in cannabis smoking). Headshops also frequently sell legal highs.

Legal highs   are drugs that do not fall under the Misuse of Drugs Act, although they may be controlled under the Medicines Act. Some are herbal (also called herbal highs) such as ephedrine, yohimbine and salvia, but some, such as poppers, are synthetic or processed. They may be sold as legal and 'safe' alternatives to illegal drugs, but are usually retailed without a licence, and are not without their own risks to health.

Needle exchange   is a harm reduction intervention enabling drug users to exchange used injecting equipment for new sterile equipment, reducing the risk of the spread of BBVs.

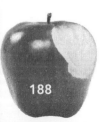

Polydrug use	is the use of more than one drug, often with the intention of enhancing or countering the effects of another drug. Polydrug use, however, may simply occur because the user's preferred drug is unavailable (or too expensive) at the time.
Problem drug use	can refer to drug use of any kind, regular or irregular, which is causing or exacerbating problems in the user's life (ie. they may experience social, financial, psychological, physical or legal problems as a result of their drug use). However, it is worth noting that when the phrase 'problem drug use' is used by UK government departments, they are usually referring to the dependent and/or chaotic use of heroin and crack cocaine, as these are the two drugs most likely to cause an individual, their family and their community the most problems.
Recreational drug use	is the use of drugs for pleasure or leisure. The term is often used to denote the use of ecstasy and other 'dance drugs', and implies that drug use has become part of someone's lifestyle (even though they may only take drugs occasionally).
Smart drugs	refers to drugs which are used to enhance cognitive abilities (such as concentration, alertness or memory). Some are stimulants – amphetamines such as Ritalin or Adderall – and some are designed to promote wakefulness, such as Modafinil, which has been used to help soldiers stay awake in battle.
Substitute prescribing	is a harm reduction intervention which aims to help people manage their withdrawal from illicit drugs. In the UK it most commonly refers to the prescription of medicines such as methadone, Subutex or buprenorphine as a way of managing withdrawal from heroin.
Tolerance	refers to the way the body gets used to the repeated presence of a drug, meaning that higher or more frequent doses are needed to maintain the same effect.
Withdrawal	is the body's reaction to the sudden absence of a drug to which it has adapted. The effects can be stopped either by taking more of the drug, by managed detoxification or by 'cold turkey' – which, depending on which drug was being used and in what quantities, may last for up to a week.

Sourced with permission from *The Media Guide to Drugs by Drugscope* at www.drugscope.org.uk/mediaguide

DrugScope is the national membership organisation for the drug sector and a leading drug information and policy charity. DrugScope has over 600 members working in the drug sector and related fields and the organisation draws on the expertise of its members to develop policy and lobby government.

For a comprehensive A–Z guide of illicit drugs and legal highs, Drugscope's *The Essential Guide to Drugs and Alcohol* e-book can be purchased from the Pavilion website at www.pavpub.com

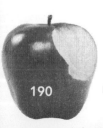

Glossary

Acetylcholine A key chemical in nerve cells formed from dietary choline that acts as a neurotransmitter and carries information on across the synapse, the space between two nerve cells.

Adenosine A chemical present in all human cells and plays an important role in energy transfer and signal transduction. It is also an inhibitory neurotransmitter.

Adiponectin A hormone produced and secreted exclusively by adipocytes (fat cells). It regulates the metabolism of lipids and glucose and influences the body's response to insulin.

Alpha-linolenic acid (ALA) An essential fatty acid found in flaxseed and walnuts that can be converted by the body into omega-3.

Amino acid The chemical units or 'building blocks' of the body that make up proteins.

Alkaloid A member of a large group of plant chemicals containing nitrogen. Many alkaloids possess potent pharmacological effects. Alkaloids include cocaine, nicotine, strychnine, caffeine, piperine, morphine, methamphetamine, mescaline, ephedrine and tryptamine.

Amphetamine ('speed') A drug with a stimulant effect on the central nervous system that can be both physically and psychologically addictive when abused.

Anaemia A deficiency in the number of red blood cells or in their haemoglobin content, resulting in pallor, shortness of breath and lack of energy.

Anaphylaxis A sudden, severe and life-threatening allergic reaction to an allergen.

Anorexia nervosa An eating disorder characterised by markedly reduced appetite or total aversion to food.

Antibody A protein (immunoglobulin) produced by lymphocytes (white blood cells) in response to an antigen.

Antigen A foreign substance that induces the production of antibodies by the immune system.

Antioxidant	Any substance that reduces oxidative damage such as that caused by 'free radicals'.
Arachidonic acid (AA)	Arachidonic acid is a polyunsaturated fatty acid present in the membrane phospholipids of body cells, and is abundant in the brain.
Atopic	An inherited tendency to develop an allergy.
Attention deficit disorder (ADD)	A development disorder that impairs one's ability to sustain focus.
Attention deficit hyperactivity disorder (ADHD)	The most common childhood-onset behavioural disorder. The core symptoms include an inability to sustain attention and concentration, developmentally inappropriate levels of activity, distractibility, and impulsivity.
Autism	A spectrum of neuropsychiatric disorders characterised by deficits in social interaction and communication, and unusual and repetitive behavior. The degree of autism varies from mild to severe in different people.
Basophil	A type of leukocyte (white blood cell) involved in inflammatory reactions in the body, especially those related to allergies and asthma. When stimulated, basophils release histamine and other enzymes that can lead to symptoms.
Bifidobacteria	A form of 'friendly' bacteria which reside in the lower part of the digestive system.
Binge eating disorder	An eating disorder characterised by periods of extreme over-eating.
Biotin	A water-soluble B-complex vitamin.
Bipolar disorder	A mood disorder sometimes called manic depression which characteristically involves cycles of depression and elation or mania.
Brain-derived neurotrophic factor (BDNF)	A protein that supports the survival of existing neurons and encourages the growth and differentiation of new neurons.
Bulimia nervosa	An eating disorder characterised by episodes of secretive excessive binge-eating followed by self-induced vomiting, abuse of laxatives and diuretics, or excessive exercise.

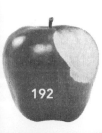

Nutrition and Addiction: A handbook © Pavilion Publishing (Brighton) Ltd 2011

Casein	The main protein found in milk and other dairy products.
Casomorphin	A particular type of protein fragment with opioid effects derived from incomplete digestion of casein.
Catecholamines	Organic compounds derived from the amino acid tyrosine that act as hormones or neurotransmitters. Examples include epinephrine (adrenaline), norepinephrine (noradrenaline) and dopamine.
Chromium	A trace element found widely in the environment and believed to influence how insulin behaves in the body.
Commensals	Normally occurring species living on or within another organism, and deriving benefit without harming or benefiting the host.
Comorbidities	Diseases or conditions that coexist with a primary disease but also stand on their own as specific diseases.
Cortisol	A hormone produced by the adrenal cortex that mediates various metabolic processes, has anti-inflammatory and immunosupressive properties, and whose levels in the blood may become elevated in response to physical or psychological stress.
Cysteine	Sulphur-containing amino acid that can be synthesized by the body. The extracellular concentration of cysteine is quite low because this amino acid typically exists in the disulfide form, cystine.
Cytokines	Small proteins released from white blood cells that act as chemical signals between cells.
Delta-6 desaturase	Enzyme that converts linoleic acid to gamma linolenic acid (GLA).
Docosahexaenoic acid (DHA)	Long-chain polyunsaturated fatty acid – a vital component of the phospholipids of human cellular membranes, especially those in the brain and retina. It is necessary for optimal development.
Digestive enzymes	Enzymes in the digestive tract which break down complex substances into simpler ones so they can be absorbed. Available in supplement form.
Dihomogamma-linolenic (DGLA)	A highly unsaturated fatty acid from the omega-6 family.

Dopamine	A major neurotransmitter present in regions of the brain that regulate movement, emotion, motivation, and the feeling of pleasure.
Dysbiosis	Humans are colonised by multitudes of commensal organisms representing members of five of the six kingdoms of life; however, our gastrointestinal tract provides residence to both beneficial and potentially pathogenic microorganisms. Imbalances in the composition of the bacterial microbiota is known as dysbiosis.
Dyslexia	A specific reading disability due to a defect in the brain's processing of graphic symbols.
Dyspraxia	A motor learning disability that affects movement and co-ordination.
Eczema	An itchy, inflammatory skin condition associated with allergy.
Eicosanoids	Signaling molecules derived from omega-3 or omega-6 fats.
Eicosapentaenoic acid (EPA)	A long-chain omega-3 fatty acid found primarily in fish and shellfish.
Endocannabinoid system	A group of neuromodulatory lipids and their receptors that are involved in a variety of physiological processes including appetite, pain-sensation, mood and memory.
Endorphin	One of the body's own painkillers, an opioid chemical produced by the body that serves to suppress pain. Endorphins are manufactured in the CNS and other parts of the body. They are released in response to neurotransmitters and bind to certain neuron receptors.
Essential fatty acid (EFA)	Unsaturated fatty acids are essential to human health and cannot be manufactured in the body.
Exorphin	Food-derived opioid peptide (ie. from gluten/dairy/soya) with morphine-like activities that may reach opiate receptors in the central nervous system and trigger their function (first described by Zioudro, Streaty and Klee in 1978).

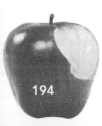

Nutrition and Addiction: A handbook © Pavilion Publishing (Brighton) Ltd 2011

Flavonoids	Water-soluble plant pigments beneficial to human health.
Folate (folic acid)	One of the B vitamins and a key factor in the synthesis of DNA and RNA.
Free radicals	Highly reactive molecules possessing unpaired electrons that are produced during metabolism of food and energy. They are believed to contribute to the molecular damage and death of body cells. They may be a factor in aging or disease.
Genotype	This is the 'internally coded, inheritable information' carried by all living organisms. This stored information is used as a 'blueprint' or set of instructions for building and maintaining a living creature. These instructions are found within almost all cells (the 'internal' part). They are written in a coded language (the genetic code), are copied at the time of cell division or reproduction and are passed from one generation to the next ('inheritable'). These instructions are intimately involved with all aspects of the life of a cell or an organism. They control everything from the formation of protein macromolecules, to the regulation of metabolism and synthesis of enzymes.
Ghrelin	A gastrointestinal hormone which appears to be a stimulant for appetite and feeding, and is considered to counterbalance the hormone leptin. Ghrelin levels increase before meals and decrease after meals.
Glutathione	A major cellular antioxidant needed for immune function and the production of energy. Glutathione is a tripeptide consisting of glutamic acid, cysteine, and glycine.
Glutamate	Amino acid that functions as the major excitatory neurotransmitter in the central nervous system.
Glutamate cystine transporter	Amino acid transport system highly specific for cystine and glutamate. Its activity is known to be induced by cystine deprivation.
Gluten	A protein found in wheat, barley or rye (oats can be contaminated with gluten).
Gluteomorphins	Peptides with opioid acitivity due to incomplete digestion of gluten.

Glycaemic index (GI)	Indicator of the ability of different types of foods that contain carbohydrate to raise blood glucose levels within two hours. Carbohydrate containing foods that break down most quickly during digestion have the highest glycaemic index.
Glycine	A non-essential amino acid and a constituent of most proteins. It functions as an inhibitory neurotransmitter in the central nervous system.
Hallucinogen	A drug that causes profound distortions in a person's perceptions of reality such as LSD.
Highly unsaturated fatty acids (HUFAs)	Special kinds of polyunsaturated fats (omega-3 and omega-6) crucial to brain development and function.
Histamine	A naturally occurring substance that is released by the immune system after being exposed to an allergen.
Homeostasis	The maintenance of a stable, constant internal environment within the body.
Hypothalamic-pituitary-adrenal axis (HPA)	A feedback loop that includes the hypothalamus, the pituitary and the adrenal glands.
Hypothalamus	Area of the brain that controls body temperature, hunger, and thirst.
Immunoglobulin (Ig)	A glycoprotein that functions as an antibody. There are five classes with different structures (IgA, IgD, IgE, IgG, IgM).
In vitro	Testing outside the body (opposite of in vivo – in the body).
Indoleamine 2, 3-dioxygenase (IDO)	A special enzyme produced in response to stress to help manage immune chemicals and to control the metabolism of tryptophan – an important amino acid in the production of the mood enhancing neurotransmitter serotonin.
Indole	Organic compound found in the amino acid tryptophan, alkaloids and pigments.
Inositol	A carbohydrate originally classed as part of the vitamin B-complex. It is required for proper formation of cell membranes. Inositol affects nerve transmission and helps in transporting fats within the body.

Insulin	A hormone made by the pancreas that controls the level of glucose in the blood. Cells cannot utilise glucose without insulin.
Isotype	Any of the subclasses of immunoglobulins produced by the immune system and defined by the chemical and antigenic characteristics of their constant regions. In humans, the five human isotypes are: IgA, IgD, IgG, IgE and IgM. IgG and IgA also have subclasses.
Ion channels	These allow the movement of ions across cell membranes; present in the membranes that surround all biological cells.
L-dopa	Amino acid that is the metabolic precursor of dopamine, is converted in the brain to dopamine, and used in synthetic form to treat Parkinson's disease.
Lactobacilli	Bacteria found in the mouth, intestinal tract and vagina. Lactobacilli also live in fermenting products, such as yogurt.
Leptin	A hormone that has a central role in fat metabolism and is expressed predominantly by adipocytes (fat cells).
Leukotrienes	Hormone-like chemicals derived from fatty acids which contribute to inflammation and allergy.
Limbic system	A network of structures in the brain involved in memory and emotions.
Linoleic acid (LA)	A polyunsaturated fatty acid of the omega-6 family abundant in many vegetable oils.
Lipid peroxidation	The oxidative degradation of lipids. The process in which 'free radicals' 'steal' electrons from the lipids in cell membranes, resulting in cell damage.
Macronutrients	Nutrients that provide calories or energy: carbohydrate, protein and fat.
Magnetic resonance imaging (MRI)	A special radiology technique designed to image internal structures of the body using magnetism, radio waves and a computer to produce the images of body structures.
Mast cells	Mast cells are an important part of the immune system response. They release inflammatory substances including histamine.

Metabolome	The complete set of molecular metabolites (eg. hormones and other signalling molecules) found in the body.
Metagenome	Most commonly refers to our own genome plus the genome of all our microbial flora.
Metaplasticity	Activity-dependent regulation of the plastic state of neurons. The view that the synapse's previous history of activity determines its current plasticity, meaning it can be moulded.
Methadone	An opioid that is used mainly to wean people off their addiction to stronger opioids such as diamorphine (heroin).
Microbiome	Microbiome is the totality of microbes, their genetic elements (genomes), and environmental interactions in a defined environment. A defined environment could, for example, be the gut of a human being or a soil sample.
Microbiota	The microorganisms that typically inhabit a bodily organ or part; flora.
Micronutrients	Needed for life in small quantities, such as vitamins, minerals, trace elements.
Monoamine	Class of hormones or neurotransmitters which have one amine eg. catecholamines (dopamine, noradrenaline) and indoleamines (serotonin, melatonin).
Monoamine transporters (MAT)	Structures in nerve-cell membranes that function as neurotransmitter transporters transferring monoamine neurotransmitters in or out of cells, such as the dopamine transporter (DAT) and the serotonin transporter (SERT).
Monounsaturated fatty acids	Fatty acids whose carbon chains have one double bond. Foods high in monounsaturated fats include canola and olive oil.
Mutualists	Originated from the Latin word *mutuus*, meaning lent, borrowed, or mutual. A relationship between two organisms where both organisms benefit. For example, bacteria that expand in the intestinal niche and provide metabolic pathways complementing the digestive functions of the host.

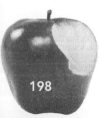

N-acetylcysteine (NAC)	Antioxidant agent derived from the amino acid cysteine. Can be used as a mucolytic agent and in the management of paracetamol (acetaminophen) overdose. Other uses include sulfate repletion where cysteine and related sulfur amino acids may be depleted.
Neuron	Nerve cell that sends and receives electrical signals.
Neuroplasticity	The brain's natural ability to form new connections in order to compensate for injury or changes in the environment. The ability of the brain to reorganise pathways between neurons as a result of new experiences.
Neurotransmitter	A substance (such as noradrenaline or acetylcholine) that transmits nerve impulses across a synapse.
NMDA receptor	The N-methyl-D-aspartate (NMDA) receptor is a type of receptor activated by the amino acid glutamate and is the predominant molecular device for controlling synaptic plasticity and memory function.
Non-communicable diseases	Chronic conditions that do not result from an acute infectious process, including cardiovascular disease, cancer, mental health problems, diabetes mellitus, chronic respiratory disease and musculoskeletal conditions.
Noradrenaline (norepinephrine)	Catecholamine neurotransmitter used by the sympathetic nervous system and the brain.
Nuclear Factor kappa B	Acts as a cellular specialist in the production of inflammation in the face of infection and certain stressors. It is a sophisticated amplifier of over 400 genes dedicated to increasing inflammation to defend us, which if not controlled can lead to inflammation-based illnesses.
Nutrimetabonomics	Nutrimetabonomics is the collection and analysis of fluids and metabolites produced by a human and its microbes after eating certain foods. It assesses the food's effects on metabolism.
Omega-3	A class of essential fatty acids found primarily in fish oils, especially from salmon and other cold-water fish. EPA (eicosapentaenoic acid) and DHA (docosahexaenoic acid) are the two principal omega-3 fatty acids.

Omega-6	A class of essential fatty acids found in seeds and nuts, and the oils extracted from them. GLA (gamma-linolenic acid) is a principle omega-6 fatty acid found primarily in hemp, borage and evening primrose oil.
Omega-9	Monounsaturated fatty acids found in olive oil and avocados. Unlike essential fatty acids they can be manufactured by the body.
Opiate	A medication or illegal drug either derived from the opium poppy, or that mimics the effect of an opiate (a synthetic opiate). Opiate drugs are narcotic sedatives that depress activity of the central nervous system, reduce pain, and induce sleep. Long-term use can produce addiction, and overuse can cause overdose and potentially death.
Opioid antagonist	A receptor antagonist acting on opioid receptors. Commonly used opioid antagonist drugs are naloxone and naltrexone, which bind to the opioid receptors but do not activate the receptors. This effectively blocks the receptor, preventing the body from responding to opiates and endorphins.
Opioid peptides	Short sequences of amino acids, which mimic the effect of opiates in the brain.
Oral allergy syndrome (OAS)	An allergic reaction in hayfever sufferers contained to the mouth and throat, resulting from direct contact with certain fruits, nuts, and vegetables. It is not usually life-threatening (unlike anaphylaxis).
Orthomolecular medicine	Linus Pauling defined orthomolecular medicine as the treatment of disease by the provision of the optimum molecular environment, especially the optimum concentrations of substances normally present in the human body.
Oxidative stress	Increased oxidant production in cells characterised by the release of 'free radicals' and resulting in cellular degeneration.
Pathobionts	Normally occurring species that due to changes in the environmental cues are seen as a threat by the immune system.

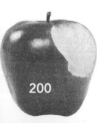

 Nutrition and Addiction: A handbook © Pavilion Publishing (Brighton) Ltd 2011

Pathophenotype	A new approach to classifying human disease that uses conventional reductionism and incorporates the non reductionist approach of systems biomedicine that takes into account the interactions of multiple systems on the human genome. Such phenotypes result from many variables with genetic makeup, physiological factors such as age, gender, stress, disease, etc., and environmental factors such as diet, lifestyle, exposure to environmental toxins and environmental history (including in utero experiences), concomitant drug and alcohol usage, and even, or perhaps especially in light of emerging experimental work in areas such as diabetes and obesity and gut microbiology.
Phenotype	This is the 'outward, physical manifestation' of the organism. These are the physical parts, the sum of the atoms, molecules, macromolecules, cells, structures, metabolism, energy utilisation, tissues, organs, reflexes and behaviours; anything that is part of the observable structure, function or behaviour of a living organism.
Phytochemicals (phytonutrients)	A large group of compounds produced by plants to protect them from toxins and environmental pollutants. Although not considered essential nutrients, they are believed to contain health protecting qualities.
Polypeptide	Amino acids make up polypeptides which in turn make up proteins.
Polyphenol	A group of chemical substances with antioxidant and anti-inflammatory properties found in berries, walnuts, olives, tea leaves, grapes and many other plants.
Potassium	An electrolyte and mineral that plays a major role in maintaining fluid and acid-base balance and assists in regulating neuromuscular activity.
Prostaglandins	Hormone-like substances required for a wide range of body functions such as the contraction and relaxation of smooth muscle, the dilation and constriction of blood vessels, control of blood pressure, and modulation of inflammation.

Proteins	Proteins consist of one or more chains of amino acids and are required for the structure, function, and regulation of the body's cells, tissues, and organs. Each protein has unique functions.
Proteomic	The term 'proteomics' was coined in 1994 by Marc Wilkins who defined it as *'the study of proteins, how they are modified, when and where they are expressed, how they are involved in metabolic pathways and how they interact with one another.'*
Psychosis	A mental illness seen primarily in schizophrenia and bipolar disorders. Symptoms include seeing, hearing, smelling or tasting things that are not there, paranoia and delusional thoughts.
Psychotropic	Referring to drugs that alter behaviour, mood, and perception.
Randomised controlled trial (RCT)	A study in which people are allocated at random to receive one of several clinical interventions. One of these interventions is the standard of comparison or control. The control may be a standard practice, a placebo ('sugar pill'), or no intervention at all. RCTs seek to measure and compare the outcomes after the participants receive the interventions. Because the outcomes are measured, RCTs are quantitative studies.
Receptor	A structure on the surface of a cell (or inside a cell) that selectively receives and binds a specific substance. In neurology, a terminal of a sensory nerve that receives and responds to stimuli.
Regulatory T cell	Specialised white blood cell that regulates the activity of another T cell. This process can be beneficial or harmful. There are several different types of regulatory T cells.
Reward deficiency syndrome	Refers to the breakdown of the reward cascade and resultant aberrant conduct due to genetic and environmental influences.
Saccharomyces boulardii	A tropical strain of yeast first isolated from lychee and mangosteen fruit. Classified as a probiotic, it is used to maintain and restore the natural gut flora in the treatment and prevention of gastrointestinal disorders.

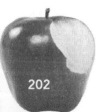

Saturated fat	Type of food fat that is solid at room temperature. Most saturated fats come from animal food products, but some plant oils, such as palm and coconut oil, also contain high levels.
Schizophrenia	A complex mental health disorder characterised by hallucinations and/or delusions, personality changes, withdrawal, and serious thought and speech disturbances.
Seasonal affective disorder (SAD)	A type of depression that tends to occur in the autumn and winter.
Secretory IgA (sIgA)	An important immunoglobulin found in the gastrointestinal tract and mucus secretions throughout the body. SIgA is our first line of defence against bacteria, food residues, fungi, parasites and viruses. Low levels are believed to be associated with allergy, autoimmune and GI diseases.
Selenium	An essential trace mineral which activates glutathione peroxidase, an antioxidant enzyme involved in the neutralisation of 'free radicals'.
Short chain fatty acids	Short chain fatty acids having a chain length up to roughly six carbon atoms long. They are produced by bacterial anaerobic fermentation, particularly of dietary carbohydrates, in the large intestine. They are readily absorbed and are metabolised in the liver and muscle tissues, producing energy and supporting tolerance through inflammation control.
Symbionts	An organism in a symbiotic relationship.
Symbiosis	Originated from the Greek words syn and biosis, meaning 'with' and 'living' coined in 1879 by the mycologist Heinrich Anton de Bary. The original meaning of symbiosis is the 'living together of unlike organisms'. Symbiosis is generally understood as a relationship between two organisms from which both organisms benefit.
Synapse	A specialised junction at which a neuron communicates with another neuron or a different target cell. The neuron releases a chemical transmitter (a neurotransmitter) that diffuses across a small gap and activates specific specialised sites called receptors situated on the target cell.

Taurine   A non-essential amino acid, but it may be essential for individuals with certain diseases or nutritional concerns.

Thromboxane   Member of the family of lipids known as eicosanoids. Causes blood clotting and constriction of blood vessels.

Thymus   An organ that is part of the lymphatic system, in which T lymphocytes grow and multiply. The thymus is in the chest behind the breastbone.

Trace elements   Nutrients required by plants, animals or humans in minute amounts.

Trans fats   A type of fat formed from hydrogenation which changes a liquid oil into a solid fat. Trans fats are found in processed foods and are now considered to be harmful to health.

Triglycerides   The chemical form in which most fat exists in food as well as in the body. Triglycerides in plasma are derived from fats eaten in foods or made in the body from other energy sources like carbohydrates. Excess levels contribute to a person's risk of heart disease.

Tryptophan   An amino acid that occurs in proteins; it is essential for growth and normal metabolism and is a precursor of niacin, serotonin and melatonin.

Tyramine   A naturally occurring compound derived from tyrosine, an amino acid. It acts as an adrenaline releasing agent; found in various foods and beverages such as cheese and red wine, and thought to trigger migraines in some people.

Unsaturated fat   A fat that is liquid at room temperature and comes from a plant such as olive, peanut, corn, cottonseed, sunflower, safflower, or soybean.